English in Medicine

A course in communication skills

Eric H. Glendinning
Beverly A. S. Holmström

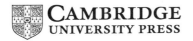

CAMBRIDGE
UNIVERSITY PRESS

Published by the Press Syndicate of the University of Cambridge
The Pitt Building, Trumpington Street, Cambridge CB2 1RP
40 West 20th Street, New York, NY 10011–4211, USA
10 Stamford Road, Oakleigh, Melbourne 3166, Australia

© Cambridge University Press 1987

This edition first published 1984
Eleventh printing 1995

Printed in Great Britain
by Scotprint Ltd, Musselburgh, Scotland

Library of Congress catalogue card number: 86–11761

British Library cataloguing in publication data

Glendinning, Eric H.

English in medicine
1. English language – Text-books for
foreign speakers   2. Medicine – Language
3. English language – Technical English
I. Title   II. Holström, Beverly A.S.
428.2′4′02461   PE1128

ISBN 0 521 31165 9 coursebook
ISBN 0 521 32332 0 cassette

Contents

Contents

Thanks

This book could not have been written without the considerable help of members of the medical profession. We acknowledge in particular the great debt we owe to Sheila Glendinning MB, ChB and Dr Alan Spence Watson for giving up so much of their precious free time to advise on medical content throughout the production of this book.

For additional help with materials and advice on case histories, warm thanks are due to Dr Evelyn Byrne MRCP, Dr Jean Braun MD, Mrs Maureen MacGregor SRN, Emeritus Professor James Walker, Rebecca Tomlinson of the BMA London, Sindy Leung, and Michael Holmström.

A special thanks is also due to Pat Coulter for typing the many drafts, to Dr Hamish Watson for his encouragement and comments on the final manuscript, and to our editor, Desmond O'Sullivan.

To the many overseas doctors, medical students, nurses and others who have worked through the successive drafts of these materials with good humour, we offer sincere thanks for all the suggestions and practical advice.

Finally, past and present teachers of the Edinburgh Language Foundation deserve our gratitude for their helpful comments. In particular we would like to thank Helen Mantell, Helen Tyrrell, Anne Rowe and Claire MacGregor.

To the reader

This book aims to help you communicate in English with patients and their relatives, with medical colleagues and with paramedical staff. It is also designed to help you cope with medical reading of all kinds from documents to journal articles. Those of you who are students will find this book useful in the clinical phase of your studies. The section on reading skills will help you with your textbooks. The authors have co-operated closely with members of the medical profession in preparing this text to ensure authenticity. They have long experience in helping overseas medical personnel with their communicative needs.

The book is divided into seven units. The units are organised in a way which mirrors your own dealings with a patient. You start with the English needed for consultations and continue with examinations – both general and specialised. Next you study the language required to discuss investigations, diagnoses and treatment both with the patient and with English-speaking colleagues. Finally you examine the English of treatment.

Each unit has four sections. The first section introduces new language and provides interesting practice activities. The second practises further language items on the same general theme and includes medical documents of different kinds. The third deals with reading skills and aims to develop the skills needed to understand a range of medical texts including hospital documents and text-books. The final section consolidates the material covered in the first two sections in the context of a continuing case history which provides a link from unit to unit.

The language activities in this book have four different labels: Task, Language focus, Practice and Role-play.

Task heads listening and reading activities designed to involve your medical knowledge in helping you to anticipate what you hear or read. The book is accompanied by a cassette which contains the recordings for the listening tasks. A complete tapescript is provided at the back of the book. Follow the instructions for each task carefully. If you are asked to predict, make sure you do the exercise before you listen to the cassette. Once the listening task is completed, you can listen to the extract as often as you like. If you are working without the cassettes, treat all the listening tasks as reading tasks and use the tapescript as your text.

Language focus draws your attention to the key language items introduced by the tasks, starting with basic questions. The focus is on the language used in medical communication, and grammar points without medical relevance are not included.

Practice covers a range of guided activities to practise and help you remember the new language items. A key and glossary are provided at the end of the book to help those studying alone.

Role-play covers freer activities intended to give you practice in asking questions, instructing and explaining. Wherever possible, work with a friend or collegue. If you work alone, always take the part of the doctor. Read both parts; then write down what you would say to the patient, relative or medical colleague.

To the teacher

This text is the product of many years' teaching. It has been used successfully both by those with long experience in Medical English and also by those new to this field. You do not require any special knowledge of medicine to use this book, but you do require an interest in the language needs of the medical professions and a grasp of the teaching techniques of the communicative approach. You provide the teaching expertise; the student provides the medical knowledge. The right blend will give results.

The organisation of the book and the objectives of each type of activity – Task, Language focus, Practice and Role-play – are outlined in the note to the reader. With a little practice, you will be able to devise other activities of your own, based on the textbook models, and using widely available sources such as medical journals. For example, a journal case history can provide practice in case-taking (Unit 2, Practice 2), scanning (Unit 1, Task 5), and is source material for a cloze exercise (Unit 6, Task 8) or a doctor–patient, doctor–relative role-play.

Many of the authentic documents used (e.g. the Discharge Summary in Unit 7) lend themselves to a variety of activities in addition to those described in the book. Be creative and you will get the most out of this text and from your teaching.

Unit 1   Taking a history I

1.1   Asking basic questions

Task 1   [cassette icon]

Study this extract from an interview between a doctor and his patient. As you listen, complete the Present Complaint section of the case notes below.

SURNAME Hall		**FIRST NAMES** Kevin	
AGE 32	**SEX** M	**MARITAL STATUS** M	
OCCUPATION Lorry driver			
PRESENT COMPLAINT			

Now compare your notes with those made by the doctor. These are given in the Key to this unit. Explain these sections in the notes.

1 a.m.
2 c/o
3 SEX   M
4 MARITAL STATUS   M
5 "Dull and throbbing" Why are these words in quote marks (" ")?
6 3/12

Language focus 1

Note how the doctor starts the interview:
— *What's brought you along today?*

Other ways of starting an interview are:
— *What can I do for you?*
— *What seems to be the problem?*

Note how the doctor asks how long the problem has lasted.
— *How long have they been bothering you?*

Another way of asking about this is:
— *How long have you had them?*

Practice 1

Study this short dialogue.

Doctor: Well, Mr Black. *What's brought you along today?*
Patient: I've got a bad dose of flu (1).
Doctor: *How long has it been bothering you?*
Patient: Two or three days (2).

Practise this dialogue, getting a friend or fellow student to play the part of the patient. He/she can select replies from lists (1) and (2) below. Use all the ways of starting an interview and asking how long the problem has lasted.

(1)	(2)
a bad dose of flu	a fortnight
terrible constipation	two or three days
swollen ankles	since Tuesday
a pain in my stomach	for almost a month

Language focus 2

Note how the doctor asks where the problem is:
– *Which part of your head is affected?*

Other ways of finding this out are:
– *Where does it hurt?* *
– *Where is it sore?* *

Note how the doctor asks about the type of pain:
– *Can you describe the pain?*

Other ways of asking this are:
– *What's the pain like?*
– *What kind of pain is it?*

---

* *Hurt* is a verb. We use it like this: *My foot hurts.*
   Sore is an adjective. We can say, *My foot is sore* or *I have a sore foot.*

Practice 2

Practise finding out these kinds of information. Work in the same way as in Practice 1. Use all the methods given in Language focus 2 in your questioning.

Doctor: *What part of your back (chest, head, etc.) is affected?*
Patient: Just here.
Doctor: *Can you describe the pain?*
Patient: It's .... (1).

(1)
a dull sort of ache
a feeling of pressure
very sore, like a knife
a burning pain

Language focus 3

Note how the doctor asks if anything relieves the pain:
– *Is there anything that makes it better?* *

Similarly he can ask:
– *Does anything make it worse?*

Doctors often ask if anything else affects the problem . For example,
– *What effect does food have?*
– *Does lying down help the pain?*

Practice 3

Work with a partner. In each of these cases, ask your partner where the pain is. Then ask two other appropriate questions to help you reach a diagnosis. A diagram showing your partner where to indicate in each case is in the Key. Use all the ways of questioning we have studied in this section. For example,

Doctor: *Where does it hurt?*
Patient: Right across here. (indicating the central chest area)
Doctor: *Can you describe the pain?*
Patient: It's like a heavy weight pressing on my chest.
Doctor: *Does anything make it better?*
Patient: If I stop for a bit, it goes away.

In this example, the patient's symptoms suggest angina.

Now try each of these four cases in the same way.

1 Doctor: ....
  Patient: Here, just under my ribs. (1)
  Doctor: ....
  Patient: It gets worse and worse. Then it goes away.
  Doctor: ....
  Patient: Food makes it worse.

* *Better* means *improved* or *relieved*. It does not mean *cured*.

2 Doctor: ....
  Patient: It's right here. (2)
  Doctor: ....
  Patient: It's a gnawing kind of pain.
  Doctor: ....
  Patient: Yes, if I eat, it gets better.

3 Doctor: ....
  Patient: Down here. (3)
  Doctor: ....
  Patient: It's a sharp, stabbing pain. It's like a knife.
  Doctor: ....
  Patient: If I take a deep breath, or I cough, it's really sore.

4 Doctor: ....
  Patient: Just here. (4)
  Doctor: ....
  Patient: My chest feels raw inside.
  Doctor: ....
  Patient: When I cough, it hurts most.

Role-play 1

Work in pairs. **A** should start.

A: Play the part of the doctor. Repeat the exercise but add two or three more questions in each case to help you decide on a diagnosis. For instance, in the example where the patient's symptoms suggest angina, you could ask:
  – *Does anything make it worse?*
  – *How long does the pain last?*
  – *Is there anything else you feel at the same time?*

B: Play the part of the patients. Use the replies in the examples and the extra information in the Key to help you.

1.2   Taking notes

Task 2

These notes show the doctor's findings when he examined Mr Hall. Note the
explanations given for the abbreviations used. What do the other ringed abbreviations stand for?

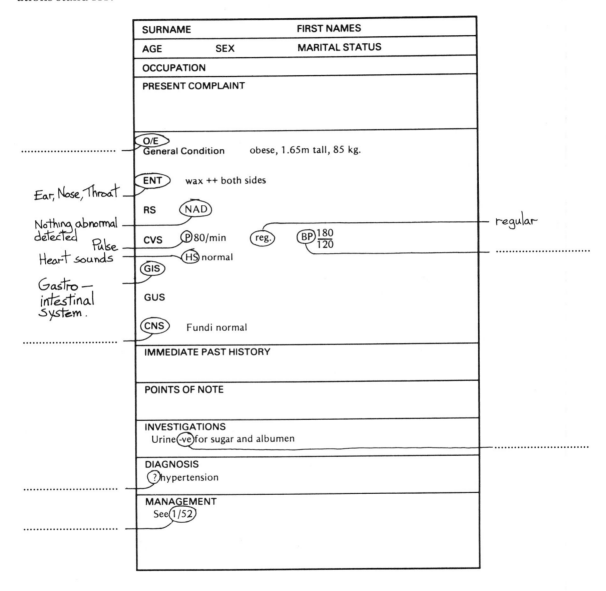

Task 3

Study this letter from a GP to a consultant. Write down the questions which a doctor might ask to obtain the information ringed in the letter. For example,

4 *How long did it last?*
8 *What was the cause of death?*

CLINICAL DETAILS

Date _____ Oct 3rd 1985 _____

Dear _____ Dr Scott _____

I would be grateful for your opinion and advice with regard to

(Name) _____ GREEN, Peter _____

URGENT
Please indicate in the box ☐

A brief outline of history, symptoms and signs and present therapy is given below:

This 42-year-old (salesman)[1] had a severe attack of (central chest pain)[2] (six months ago)[3] which (lasted 10 mins)[4] and was (relieved by rest.)[5] This has recurred several times (after exertion.)[6] His father (died aged 56)[7] of a (coronary thrombosis.)[8] Physical examination was normal and I refer him to you for further assessment in view of his age.

Diagnosis:- angina

Thank you for seeing him

Yours sincerely,

If transport required please state:
Stretcher/Sitting case
Sitting case – two man lift

☒YES ☐NO

Signature *William Keeble Jones*

Task 4 🗩

Listen to the interview between the hospital consultant and Mr Green. Complete the consultant's notes. The information in the letter will also be useful. Use the abbreviations you have studied in this section and in 1.1.

SURNAME .... (1)	**FIRST NAMES** Peter

AGE .... (2) **SEX** M	**MARITAL STATUS** M	

OCCUPATION .... (3)

PRESENT COMPLAINT
.... (4) chest pain radiating to L arm. Started with severe attack c̄ dyspnoea. Pain lasted .... (5) relieved by rest. Has occurred since on exertion.

O/E
General Condition

ENT

RS   Chest .... (6)

CVS   .... (7)   70/min   .... (8) 130/80
.... (9)   normal
GIS

GUS

CNS

IMMEDIATE PAST HISTORY

POINTS OF NOTE

INVESTIGATIONS

DIAGNOSIS

Practice 4

Study these case notes. What questions might the doctor have asked to obtain the information they contain?

a)

SURNAME James	FIRST NAMES Robert

AGE 48 **SEX** M **MARITAL STATUS** S

OCCUPATION Builder

PRESENT COMPLAINT
^c/o frontal headache 4/7 following cold.
Worse in a.m. and when bending down.
Also ^c/o being "off colour" and feverish.

POINTS OF NOTE
Analgesics c̄ some relief.

b)

SURNAME Warner **FIRST NAMES** Mary Elizabeth

AGE 34 **SEX** F **MARITAL STATUS** D

OCCUPATION Housewife

PRESENT COMPLAINT ^c/o episodic headaches many years,
lasting 1-2 days every 3-4 months. Pain behind eyes c̄ nausea.
"tightness" back of head.
Depressed c̄ pain, interfering c̄ housework.

Role-play 2

Work in pairs and try to recreate the consultation. **A** should start.

A: Play the part of the patients. Use the case notes as prompts.
B: Play the part of the doctor. Find out what the patient is complaining of. Do not look at the case notes.

1.3 Reading skills: scanning a case history

Task 5

Find and underline this information about the patient as quickly as you can.
Number the information in the margin.

1 age
2 symptoms at the onset of his present illness
3 state when found by his landlady
4 why he consulted his GP five years earlier
5 significant findings on that occasion
6 diagnosis made when referred to hospital
7 health over the last five years
8 alcohol consumption

A 63-YEAR OLD bachelor who worked as a bank clerk developed symptoms similar to those which had affected several of his colleagues who had been diagnosed as having influenza. He felt feverish, had a running nose, aches in his muscles and generalized malaise. He therefore stayed off work in his bed-sitting room. After 48 hours the landlady noticed that the milk on the doorstep had not been taken in for the previous two days, and also that his cat had not been fed. On entering his room she found him confused and delirious. She called a doctor, who immediately had him admitted to hospital.

The only significant history was that five years previously, when he had last consulted his general practitioner because of bleeding haemorrhoids, a routine blood count had been performed which showed Hb 12.6 g/dl with normal film, and white count 21,000/mm³ (21×10^9/l), 90 per cent of which were lymphocytes. At that stage he was referred to hospital, where it was found that he had some enlarged lymph nodes in both sides of the neck and both axillae, and that the spleen tip was palpable. Chronic lymphatic leukaemia was diagnosed. The patient was kept under six-monthly follow-up, with no change in the signs or blood picture. He had remained asymptomatic throughout the five-year period.

In the personal history, his weight had been steady and his bowels were now less troublesome since he had taken bran each morning which had a good effect. He smoked 30 cigarettes a day but only drank moderately.

1.4   Case history: William Hudson

Task 6   🔲

In this section in each unit we will follow the medical history of William Hudson. In this extract he is visiting his new doctor for the first time. As you listen, complete the personal details and Present Complaint section of the case notes below.

SURNAME Hudson		FIRST NAMES William Henry
AGE	**SEX**	**MARITAL STATUS**
OCCUPATION		
PRESENT COMPLAINT		
O/E **General Condition**		
ENT		
RS		
CVS		
GIS		
GUS		
CNS		
IMMEDIATE PAST HISTORY		

Role-play 3   👥

Work in pairs. Try to recreate the consultation. **A** should start.

A: Play the part of William Hudson. Use the notes to help you.
B: Play the part of the doctor.

The case of William Hudson continues in 2.4.

Unit 2   Taking a history II

2.1   Asking about systems

Task 1

Listen to this extract from an interview between a doctor and her patient. The patient is a 50-year-old housewife who has complained of feeling tired, lacking energy and not being herself. As you listen, show whether the patient has or has not a significant complaint by marking the appropriate column with a tick (✓) for each system.

System	Complaint	No complaint	Order
ENT			
RS			
CVS			
GIS			1
GUS			
CNS			
Psychiatric			

Task 2

Listen again and number the order in which the above information is obtained. The first one is marked for you.

Language focus 1

Note how the doctor asks about the systems:
— *Have you any trouble with* your stomach or bowels?
— *Any problems with* your waterworks?
— *What about* coughs or wheezing or shortness of breath?
— *What's* your appetite *like*?
— *Have you noticed* any weakness or tingling in your limbs?

Practice 1

Now match each of the suspected problems in the first column with a suitable question from the second column. For example, 1 = c.

Suspected problem	*Question*
1 depression	a) Have you had any pain in your chest?
2 cardiac failure	b) Do you ever get wheezy?
3 asthma	c) What sort of mood have you been in recently?
4 prostate	d) Any problem with your waterworks?
5 coronary thrombosis	e) Have you ever coughed up blood?
6 cancer of the lung	f) Have you had any shortness of breath?

Role-play 1

Work in pairs. **A** should start.

A: Play the part of a doctor. Ask questions about systems and specific problems for each of these cases. The patient has enough information to answer at least two key questions.
B: Play the part of the patients. Your problems are given in the Key.

1 The patient is a man in late middle-age. He has coughed up blood several times in the last few weeks.
2 The patient is an elderly man. He has been getting more and more constipated over the past few months.
3 The patient is a middle-aged woman. She gets pain in her stomach after meals.
4 The patient is a young woman. She has pain when she is passing urine.
5 The patient is a young man. He has a frontal headache.

When you have finished, look in the Key at the diagnosis for each case. Match the diagnoses to the patients by numbering them 1 to 5.

2.2   Asking about symptoms

Task 3   [cassette icon]

In this extract a physician interviews a patient who has been admitted to hospital suffering from FUO (fever of unknown origin). The physician suspects TB. He has already asked about family history, etc. The form below is part of an FUO checklist. First listen and tick (✓) each point covered in the interview.

Now listen again to indicate the order in which the points are covered by writing a number in the correct box. For example, *duration* is covered first, so write 1 in that box.

FEVER	duration	1	chills	
	frequency		sweats	
	time		night sweats	
			rigor	

GENERAL SYMPTOMS	malaise		wt loss		anorexia	
	weakness		drowsiness		vomiting	
	myalgia		delirium		photophobia	

	bleeding?		nose	
			skin	
			urine	

ACHES AND PAINS	head		abdomen		loin	
	teeth		chest		back	
	eyes		neck		pubic	

	muscle	
	joints	
	bone	

SKIN	rash			**CVS**	dyspnoea	
	pruritis				palpitations	
	bruising				ht irregularity	

GIS	diarrhoea			**RESPIRATORY**	cough	
	melaena				coryza	
					sore throat	
					dyspnoea	

URINARY	dysuria				pleuritic pain	
	frequency				sputum	
	strangury				haemoptysis	
	discolouration	

NEURO-LOGICAL	vision	
	photophobia	
	blackouts	
	diplopia	

Practice 2

Study this extract from a case history.

The patient was a 59-year-old man, *head of a small engineering firm* (1), who *complained of central chest pain* (2) which occurred *on exertion* (3) and was *sometimes accompanied by sweating* (4). He *smoked 40 cigarettes a day* (5). The pain had *first appeared three months previously* (6) and was *becoming increasingly frequent* (7). He had noticed some *weight gain recently (4 kg)* (8) and also complained that his hair had become very dull and lifeless. He felt the cold much more than he used to. He *denied any palpitations* (9) or *ankle oedema* (10).

What questions might a doctor ask a patient to obtain the information in italics in the case history? Use the question types studied in Unit 1 and this unit. You may ask more than one question for each piece of information. For example,

1 What's your job?
2 What's brought you along today? Which part of your chest is affected?

When you have finished, put your questions in the most natural order for a consultation.

Role-play 2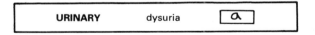

Work in pairs. **A** should start.

A: Play the part of the patient. Base your replies on the information given in the extract above.
B: Play the part of the doctor. Find out what the patient is complaining of.

Task 4

Here are some other questions which might be asked to a patient complaining of FUO. Which problems in the checklist in Task 3 do they refer to? Indicate on the form by writing the appropriate letter in the correct box.

Example: a) Have you any pain in passing water?

URINARY	dysuria	a

b) Do you suffer from double vision?
c) Any shortness of breath?
d) Does light bother you?
e) Are your stools black?
f) Do you have a cold?

Language focus 2

Listen again to the FUO extract from Task 3. Note that the doctor uses rising intonation for these questions.
- *Any pain in your muscles?*
- *Have you lost any weight?*
- *Have you had a cough at all?*
- *Is there any blood in it?*
- *Have you had any pains in your chest?*

When we ask Yes/No questions like these, we normally use rising intonation. Note that the voice changes on the important word. For example,

- Any pain in your *muscles?*

Underline the important word in each of the questions above. Then listen again to see if you can hear the change on these words. Check your answers with the Key.

Practice 3

Match each of the medical terms for common symptoms in column 1 with a term which a patient would easily understand or might use, from column 2. For example, 1 = k.

1	*2*
1 paraesthesia	a) swelling, puffiness
2 productive cough	b) indigestion
3 anaesthesia	c) coughing up phlegm or spit
4 restrosternal chest pain	d) trouble holding your water
5 orthopnea	e) cramp in the leg muscles which comes and goes
6 stress incontinence	f) numbness
7 dysmenorrhoea	g) sleeplessness
8 dyspepsia	h) out of breath, out of puff, breathlessness
9 oedema	i) painful periods
10 intermittent claudication	j) pain behind the breast bone
11 insomnia	k) pins and needles
12 dyspnoea	l) shortness of breath when you lie down

Role-play 3

Work in pairs. **B** should start.

A: Play the part of a patient. Use the notes in the Key to help you.

B: Play the part of the doctor. Try to find out what the patient's problems are. Remember your patient will not understand medical terms. Remember also to use rising intonation for Yes/No questions. Record your findings in the Present Complaint section of the form opposite.

When you have finished, **A** should check the doctor's notes. **B** should compare his/her notes with the Key.

SURNAME	Wilson	FIRST NAMES	Peter	

AGE	48	SEX	M	MARITAL STATUS	M

OCCUPATION	Steelrope worker

PRESENT COMPLAINT

Task 5

This is part of a letter of referral from a doctor to a consultant concerning the same patient. Using your case notes, complete this section of the letter. Use the appropriate medical terms.

Letter of referral (part 1)

```
Dear Dr MacPherson,

I'd be pleased to have your advice on the future management of this
48-year-old steelrope worker who gives a history of ........................... (1)
on exertion of one year's duration and a ........................... (2)
cough which he has had over the years.

During the last three weeks he has had three attacks of chest
tightness and pain radiating into the upper right arm. The attacks
have come on after exertion and have lasted several minutes. He has
noticed ankle ........................... (3)  increasing during the day and
relieved by overnight rest. He also gives a month's history of
........................... (4) of the right leg relieved by rest. Last
night he had an attack of acute ........................... (5) chest pain
lasting 15 minutes, associated with extreme restlessness and a
........................... (6) spit.

He gives a history of good health but had childhood whooping cough
and a wheezy bronchitis. He smokes an average of 20 to 30 cigarettes
a day. His sister had a history of possible pulmonary tuberculosis
and his father died of a heart attack at the age of 56.
```

Task 6

Study these findings on examination and details of the treatment given. Then complete the letter of referral.

SURNAME Wilson	**FIRST NAMES** Peter
AGE 48 **SEX** M	**MARITAL STATUS** M

OCCUPATION   Steelrope worker

PRESENT COMPLAINT Retrosternal chest pain last night radiating to neck and R arm. Duration 15 mins. Accompanied by restlessness.
Diff. sleeping. Cough $\bar{c}$ rusty spit.
1 yr SOBOE, productive cough some years, past 3/52 tightness in chest x3, pain radiating to R arm, occurred on exertion, lasted mins.
Also ^{c}/o puffy ankles in the evening, intermittent claudication R calf for 1/12.

O/E
General Condition   Short, barrel-chested, orthopnea and peripheral cyanosis, early finger clubbing.

ENT

RS   Poor resp. movt. Generalised hyper-resonance.
Loss of liver dullness. Bilateral basal creps.

CVS   P 84 reg. BP 140/92 sitting. Oedema up to knees.
Sacral oedema +. JVP ↑Apex beat outside MCL in 6th L interspace.
HS I, II faint. No peripheral pulses below popliteals.

GIS   Liver palpable and tender.   2fb

GUS

CNS

MANAGEMENT
R_X aminophylline IV 250 mg over 10 mins
frusemide 20 mg IV
morphine tartrate / cyclizine tartrate 15 mg IM

Letter of referral (part 2)

On examination, he is of .... (7) build with a
barrel-shaped chest. He is .... (8) with some
peripheral .... (9) . There is also early finger
.... (10) . Pulse rate was 84, ... (11)
in time and force. BP 140/92 sitting. He has pitting
.... (12) at the ankles to the level of the knee.
There is also .... (13) sacral oedema. He has raised
jugular .... (14) pressure.

On examination of his chest, he had poor respiratory movement, some
hyper-resonance and loss of liver dullness. His apex beat was just
outside the left-mid .... (15) line in the sixth left
interspace. .... (16) sounds were closed but faint.
He also had bilateral basal .... (17) while the liver
seemed enlarged two finger breadths below the .... (18)
costal margin and somewhat tender. The peripheral pulses in the lower
limbs were impalpable below the popliteal arteries. He was given
250mg aminophylline .... (19) at 3 a.m. over
10 minutes followed by frusemide, 20mg IV, with good effect in
relieving his breathlessness. Morphine tartrate /
cyclizine tartrate, 15mg was given .... (20) at 3.15 a.m.

Yours sincerely,

Role-play 4

Work in pairs. **A** should start.

A: Play the part of a trainee doctor. Ask about the findings on examination
and treatment to date of Mr Wilson.

B: Play the part of the doctor who has examined Mr Wilson. Supply any information on Mr Wilson's examination and treatment using the notes given in
Task 6.

Task 7   🔲

Listen to this discussion between a doctor and a hospital doctor and complete the case notes given below.

SURNAME	**FIRST NAMES**
AGE **SEX**	**MARITAL STATUS**
OCCUPATION	
PRESENT COMPLAINT	
O/E **General Condition** **ENT** **RS** **CVS** **GIS** **GUS** **CNS**	
IMMEDIATE PAST HISTORY	
POINTS OF NOTE	
INVESTIGATIONS	
DIAGNOSIS	
MANAGEMENT	

Task 8   🔲

This is a transcript of the conversation between the two doctors. Try to complete the hospital doctor's questions. Then check your answers by listening to the cassette.

D: Hello, Jim. I wonder if you could see a patient for me?

HD: Certainly, John. ....(1) the story?

D: Well, it's a Mr Alan Jameson, a 53-year-old carpenter. He's been an infrequent attender in the past but he came to see me this morning complaining of *pain in his right leg and in his back* (a).

HD: And ....(2) ....(3) this start?

D: Well, *it came on about six weeks ago* (b) and it's become gradually more severe over the past couple of weeks.

HD: ....(4) the pain localised?

D: No. Poorly. At first he thought he'd just pulled a muscle. But it's got so bad that he hasn't been able to do his work properly. It's also been getting to the stage where the *pain is waking him up at night* (c), it's been so severe, and he's *also noticed some tingling in his right foot* (d). *He's having difficulty in carrying on with his work* (e). He's *also lost three kilos* (f) and has become quite depressed.

HD: ....(5) he ....(6) anything similar ....(7) the past?

D: No, not exactly, but *he has suffered from intermittent pain in his back* (g). *Paracetamol gave some relief* (h) but didn't solve the problem completely.

HD: Apart from ....(8), any ....(9) problems ....(10) health ....(11) the past?

D: No, perfectly OK.

HD: ....(12) you ....(13) anything else ....(14) examination?

D: Yes, as well as the pain he has numbness in his toes on the right foot.

Task 9

Look at the information in italics in the transcript above. What questions might a doctor ask to obtain this kind of information from a patient? For example,

... it came on about six weeks ago (b)
Question: When did you first notice the pain?

Now try the other examples (a) to (h) in the same way. In which department do you think the hospital doctor works?

2.3   Reading skills: noting information from a textbook

Task 10

Try to complete the table below which shows some of the key features of two medical problems. Then study the textbook extracts opposite to check your answers and to complete the table to help you make a differential diagnosis between the two problems.

	Angina	*Pericarditis*
Site		retrosternal or across the chest
Radiation		
Duration	few minutes only	several hours
Precipitating factors		
Relief of pain		
Accompanying symptoms		

ANGINA PECTORIS

Angina pectoris is a clinical syndrome resulting from transient myocardial ischemia. The various diseases that result in myocardial ischemia as well as the numerous pain syndromes that may be confused with angina are discussed in Chap. 4. Approximately four-fifths of all patients with angina pectoris are men, and an even larger fraction of those younger than 50 years of age are men. The typical patient is in his fifties or early sixties and seeks medical advice because of chest discomfort. The patient commonly declines to apply the word *pain* to his chest symptoms, may have difficulty describing the sensation, and will usually select words such as heaviness, pressure, smothering, tightness, choking, or squeezing. The typical discomfort is substernal in location, but other sites are also commonly involved (see below). The most important diagnostic feature of angina pectoris is its relation to exertion or emotion and its relief by rest. The discomfort comes on during physical or emotional stress, anger, fright, hurrying, or sexual activity.

The threshold for the development of angina varies with the time of day more than from day to day. The typical patient may have to stop at exactly the same spot on his way to work each morning, yet by midday he may be able to cover many times that distance without discomfort. Symptoms which develop soon after arising are common, and the patient may not be able to shave without stopping; yet he may perform moderately heavy manual labor later in the day after he has "warmed up."

Manual chores which have been performed for many years may be well tolerated, whereas unfamiliar tasks requiring comparable effort may cause angina. This pattern is commonly observed in a laborer who is asymptomatic at work but notices chest discomfort with household or recreational activities. Relatively nonstressful activities which require the hands to be held at or above the level of the head (combing hair, shaving) frequently cause symptoms in patients who are asymptomatic while performing more strenuous chores which do not require elevation of the arms. This phenomenon is thought to be related to the increased total body oxygen requirements associated with continuous contraction of the antigravity muscles of the arms and shoulder girdles. The pain may occur during or after eating. Exposure to cold temperature or to wind may accentuate or precipitate the symptoms. Coronary spasm may play a particularly important role in patients in whom the anginal threshold varies considerably.

Variation in the location and character of the discomfort may occur, and so angina pectoris should not be ruled out just because the location of the pain is atypical, especially if there is a strong relation to exertion. Myocardial ischemia may be characterized by pain in the neck, jaw, throat, back, shoulder, abdomen, or arm, with no symptoms in the chest. Radiation to the arms, particularly the ulnar aspect of the left arm, is common in typical angina, and sometimes the only discomfort may be in the arms or wrists, where it is often described as numbness or heaviness. Sharp pains of brief duration and prolonged dull aches localized to the left submammary area are rarely due to myocardial ischemia, but the words *knife-like* and *cutting* are occasionally utilized to describe angina.

ACUTE PERICARDITIS

Pain, a pericardial friction rub, electrocardiographic changes, and pericardial effusion with cardiac tamponade and paradoxic pulse are cardinal manifestations of many forms of acute pericarditis and will be considered prior to a discussion of the most common varieties.

Pain is an important but not invariable symptom in various forms of acute pericarditis; it is usually present in the acute infectious types and in many of the forms presumed to be related to hypersensitivity or autoimmunity. Pain is often absent in a slowly developing tuberculous, postirradiation, neoplastic or uremic pericarditis. The pain of pericarditis is often severe; its character and location have been described in Chap. 4. It is characteristically in the center of the chest, referred to the back and the trapezius ridge. Often the pain is pleuritic, i.e., sharp and aggravated by inspiration, coughing, and changes in body position, but occasionally it is a steady, constrictive pain, which radiates into either arm or both arms and resembles that of myocardial ischemia; confusion with myocardial infarction is common. Characteristically, however, the pain is relieved by sitting up and leaning forward. This problem becomes even more perplexing when, with acute pericarditis, the serum transaminase level rises to about 80 units. However, the MB isoenzyme of creatine kinase does not rise in acute pericarditis.

The *pericardial friction rub* is the most important physical sign; it may have up to three components per cardiac cycle, as described in Chap. 248, and can sometimes be elicited only when firm pressure with the diaphragm of the stethoscope is applied to the chest wall. It is heard most frequently during expiration, but an independent pleural friction rub may be audible during inspiration, with the patient leaning forward or in the left lateral decubitus position. The rub is likely to be inconstant and transitory, and a loud to-and-fro leathery sound may disappear within a few hours, possibly to reappear the following day.

2.4   Case history: William Hudson

Task 11   🔲

Listen to this extract from a consultation with Mr Hudson. The doctor has not seen him for seven years. He has just retired from the Post Office. As you listen, complete the Present Complaint section of the case notes below.

SURNAME Hudson	FIRST NAMES William Henry
AGE SEX	MARITAL STATUS
OCCUPATION	
PRESENT COMPLAINT	

Task 12   🔲

Here is an edited version of the consultation. Complete the doctor's questions. Then check your answers with the cassette and the Tapescript.

D: Good morning. Just have a seat. I haven't seen you for a long time. ....(1)'s brought you here today?
P: Well, doctor, I've been having these headaches and I've lost a bit of weight.
D: And how long ....(2) the headaches ....(3) bothering you?
P: Well, for quite a while now. The wife passed away four months ago. I've been feeling a bit down since then.
D: ....(4) part of your head is affected?
P: Just here, on the top. It feels like a heavy weight pressing down on me.
D: ....(5) they affected your eyesight at all?
P: No, I wouldn't say so.
D: They ....(6)n't made you ....(7) sick?
P: No.
D: Now you told me you've lost some weight. ....(8)'s your appetite ....(9) like?
P: I've been off my food.
D: ....(10) about your bowels, ...(11) problems?
P: No, I'm quite all right.
D: What ....(12) your waterworks?
P: Well, I've been having problems getting started and I have to get up two or three times at night.
D: ....(13) this ....(14) on recently?
P: No, I've noticed it gradually over the past few months.
D: ....(15) pain when you ....(16) water?
P: No.
D: ....(17) you ....(18) any blood?
P: No.

Note how the actual consultation on the cassette differs slightly from this version. What differences can you note? This consultation continues in 3.4.

Unit 3   Examining a patient

3.1   Giving instructions

Task 1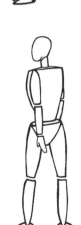

Mr Jameson (see 2.2) was examined by a neurologist. Study these drawings which show some of the movements examined. Predict the order in which the neurologist examined his patient by numbering the drawings. Drawing (e) shows the first movement examined.
Now listen to the extract from the neurologist's examination and check your predictions.

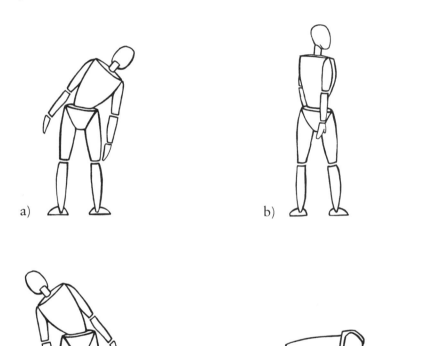

a)

b)

c)

d)

e)

f)

Language focus 1

Note how the doctor instructs the patient what to do:
– *Keep* your knees and feet steady.
– Now *I just want to see you* standing.
– *Could* you bend down as far as you can?

Instructions, especially to change position or remove clothing, are often made like this:
– Now *I would like you* to lean backwards.
– *Would you* slip off your top things, please?

The doctor often prepares the patient for the next part of the examination in this way:
– *I'm just going to* find out where the sore spot is.

Task 2

These drawings show a doctor testing a patient's reflexes. Predict the order in which the reflexes were tested by numbering them.
Now listen to the extract and check your predictions.

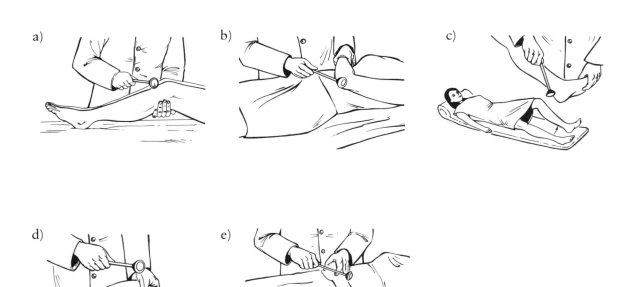

a)

b)

c)

d)

e)

Practice 1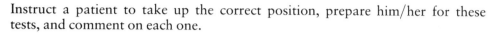

Using the pictures in Task 2 to help you, write down what you would say to a patient to test these reflexes. When you have finished, compare your instructions and comments with those on the cassette.

Practice 2

Instruct a patient to take up the correct position, prepare him/her for these tests, and comment on each one.

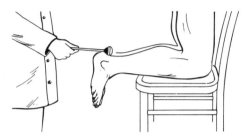

1 alternative method of eliciting the ankle jerk

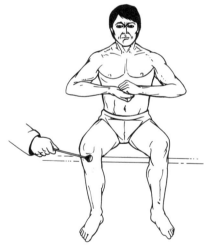

2 reinforcement in eliciting the knee jerk

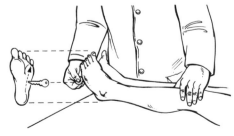

3 eliciting the plantar reflex

31

Task 3 🔲

The neurologist carries out stretch tests on Mr Jameson for the sciatic and posterior tibial nerves and the femoral nerve. Complete the gaps in his instructions with the help of the drawings below.

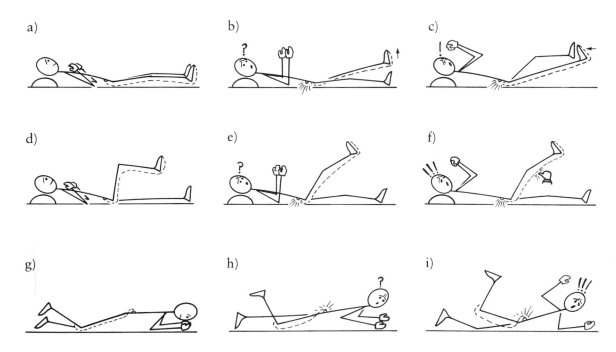

a)   b)   c)

d)   e)   f)

g)   h)   i)

D: Would you like to get onto the couch and ....(1) on your back, please? I'm going to take your left leg and see how far we can ....(2) it. Keep the knee straight. Does that hurt at all?

P: Yes, just a little. Just slightly.

D: Can I do the same with this leg? How far will this one go? Not very far. Now let's see what happens if I ....(3) your toes back.

P: Oh, that's worse.

D: I'm going to ....(4) your knee. How does that feel?

P: A little better.

D: Now let's see what happens when we ....(5) your leg again.

P: That's sore.

D: I'm just going to ....(6) behind your knee.

P: Oh, that hurts a lot.

D: Where does it ....(7)?

P: In my back.

D: Now would you ....(8) over on to your tummy? Bend your right knee. How does that ....(9)?

P: It's a little bit sore.

D: Now I'm going to ....(10) your thigh off the couch.

P: Oh, that really hurts.

Task 4

A doctor has been called as an emergency to see a 55-year-old man at home with a history of high blood pressure who has collapsed with a sudden crushing central chest pain radiating to the back and legs. List what you would examine with such a patient.

Listen to the extract and note what the doctor examined. Compare your list with the examinations carried out by the doctor.

Language focus 2

Note how the doctor marks the stages of his examination by the way his voice falls, by pauses, and by the use of expressions such as *Fine, Right, OK, That's it, Mm*.

Practice 3

Turn back to Task 3. Using the diagrams to help you, write down what you would say to a patient when making this examination.

3.2 Understanding diagrams and documents

Task 5

Study this checklist for the first examination of a patient on attendance at an
antenatal clinic. Some of these examinations are carried out as routine on subsequent visits. Mark them with a tick (✓) on the checklist.

THE FIRST EXAMINATION

1 Height
2 Weight
3 Auscultation of heart and lungs
4 Examination of breasts and nipples
5 Examination of urine
6 Examination of pelvis
7 Examination of legs
8 Inspection of teeth
9 Estimation of blood pressure
10 Blood sample for blood group
11 Blood sample for haemoglobin
12 Blood sample for serological test for syphilis
13 Blood sample for rubella antibodies
14 Examination of abdomen to assess size of uterus
15 Examination of vagina and cervix

Now study these extracts from an obstetrician's examination of a patient attending for her 32-week antenatal appointment. Match each extract to the numbered
examinations on the checklist. For example,

a) *Have you brought your urine sample?*   *5*
b) *Now would you like to sit up and I'll take your blood pressure?*
c) *Just slip off your coat and I'll check your weight next.*
d) *Now I'll take a sample of blood to check your haemoglobin.*
e) *Have you noticed any swelling of your ankles? . . . Let's have a quick look.*
f) *Now if you'd like to lie down on the couch, I'll take a look at the baby.*
   I'll just measure to see what height it is.

Task 6

Put these extracts in the order in which you would prefer to carry out these
examinations.

Role-play 1

Work in pairs. **A** should start.

A: Play the part of the obstetrician. Below are the findings on examination of a patient attending for her 32-week appointment. Base your comments to the patient on these findings.
B: Play the part of the patient. You are attending for your 32-week appointment. You are concerned about your baby. Ask the doctor if it is all right. Ask what the doctor means by a scan or any other investigation advised.

When you have completed your role-play, compare your version with what is suggested in the Key.

ANTENATAL No.

N.B. If there is anything on this card which you do not understand, do not hesitate to ask your Doctor or Midwife.

L.M.P.	? 22/3/83	Age	26
E.D.D.	1 3/2/84	Parity	O + O
	2	Height	1.55
F.M.F.F.		Blood Group	O Rh +ve

Pregnancy Test:
Date Result
1. 4/5/83 +ve
2.

Ultrasound Scans

	Date	BPD	Weeks
1			
2			
3			

Surname Wallace
First Names Mary
Address 4 Waverley Park
Wellington

Date	Wks.	Weight (kg)	Urine P	Urine S	BP	Fundus (cm.) Girth	Pres.	Level	FHH	Hb	Oed.	Problems, Investigations, Treatment etc (Please record all medicines)	Return Visit Date	Return Visit Place	G.P. Copy Sent
14/7/83	11	78.9			125/90	N.P.				12.6					
16/8/83	16	79			120/80	16									
4/10/83	22	80.7			110/80	22						AFP 16 wks. (Yes) No FMF 3/52 ago 18/8/83 Result normal			
8/11/83	26	83.5			120/80	28	Capt.		✓						
29/12/83	32	87.5			124/80	29	C	NE	✓	12.4		wt increase ++, small for dates, ref. for scan			

Analgesia	Signature	Special Problems	FOR OFFICE USE

3.3 Reading skills: using a pharmacology reference

Task 7

Using the prescribing information opposite, choose the most appropriate antibiotic for these patients.

1 A 4-year-old boy with meningitis due to pneumococcus. He is allergic to penicillin.
2 A 67-year-old man with a history of chronic bronchitis now suffering from pneumonia. The causative organism is resistant to tetracycline.
3 A 27-year-old woman with urinary tract infection in early pregnancy. She complains of nausea.
4 A 4-year-old girl with septic arthritis due to haemophilus influenzae.
5 An 18-year-old man with left leg amputation above the knee following a road traffic accident.
6 A 50-year-old woman with endocarditis caused by strep. viridans.
7 A 13-year-old girl with disfiguring acne.
8 An 8-year-old boy with tonsilitis due to β-haemolytic streptococcus.
9 A 43-year-old dairyman with brucellosis.
10 A 4-year-old unimmunised sibling of a 2-year-old boy with whooping cough.

AMPICILLIN

Indications: urinary-tract infections, otitis media, chronic bronchitis, invasive salmonellosis, gonorrhoea
Cautions; Contra-indications; Side-effects: see under Benzylpenicillin (section 5.1.1.1); also erythematous rashes in glandular fever and chronic lymphatic leukaemia; reduce dose in renal impairment. Drug interactions: see Appendix 1 (section 7)
Dose: by mouth, 0.25–1 g every 6 hours, at least 30 minutes before food
Gonorrhoea, 2 g as a single dose with probenecid 1 g; repeated for women
Urinary-tract infections, 500 mg every 8 hours
By intramuscular injection or intravenous injection or infusion, 500 mg every 4–6 hours; higher doses in meningitis
CHILD, any route, ½ adult dose

BENZYLPENICILLIN
(Penicillin G)
Indications: tonsillitis, otitis media, erysipelas, streptococcal endocarditis, meningococcal and pneumococcal meningitis, prophylaxis in limb amputation
Cautions: history of allergy; renal impairment
Contra-indications: penicillin hypersensitivity
Side-effects: sensitivity reactions including urticaria, fever, joint pains; angioedema; anaphylactic shock in hypersensitive patients; diarrhoea after administration by mouth
Dose: by intramuscular injection, 300–600 mg 2–4 times daily; CHILD up to 12 years, 10–20 mg/kg daily; NEONATE, 30 mg/kg daily
By intravenous infusion, up to 24 g daily
By intrathecal injection, 6–12 mg daily
Prophylaxis in dental procedures and limb amputation, section 5.1, Table 2

CO-TRIMOXAZOLE
A mixture of sulphamethoxazole 5 parts, trimethoprim 1 part
Indications: invasive salmonellosis, typhoid fever, bone and joint infections due to *H. influenzae*, urinary-tract infections, sinusitis, exacerbations of chronic bronchitis, gonorrhoea in penicillin-allergic patients
Cautions: blood counts in prolonged treatment, maintain adequate fluid intake, renal impairment, breast-feeding; photosensitivity. Elderly patients (see notes above). Drug interactions: see Appendix 1 (sections *2.8B, 4.8, 6.1, 8, 15*)
Contra-indications: pregnancy, infants under 6 weeks, renal or hepatic failure, jaundice, blood disorders
Side-effects: nausea, vomiting, rashes, erythema multiforme, epidermal necrolysis, eosinophilia, agranulocytosis, granulocytopenia, purpura, leucopenia; megaloblastic anaemia due to trimethoprim
Dose: by mouth, 960 mg every 12 hours, increased to 1.44 g in severe infections; 480 mg every 12 hours if treated for more than 14 days; CHILD, every 12 hours, 6 weeks to 5 months, 120 mg; 6 months to 5 years, 240 mg; 6–12 years, 480 mg
Gonorrhoea, 1.92 g every 12 hours for 2 days, or 2.4 g followed by a further dose of 2.4 g after 8 hours
By intramuscular injection or intravenous infusion, 960 mg every 12 hours
Note: 480 mg of co-trimoxazole consists of sulphamethoxazole 400 mg and trimethoprim 80 mg

ERYTHROMYCIN

Indications: alternative to penicillin in hypersensitive patients; sinusitis, diphtheria and whooping cough prophylaxis; legionnaires' disease; chronic prostatitis

Cautions: hepatic impairment. Drug interactions: see Appendix 1 (sections *2.8B, 3, 4.7, 4.8*)

Contra-indications: estolate contra-indicated in liver disease

Side-effects: nausea, vomiting, diarrhoea after large doses

Dose: by mouth, 250–500 mg every 6 hours; CHILD, 125–250 mg every 6 hours
Syphilis, 20 g in divided doses over 10 days

By slow intravenous injection or infusion, 2 g daily in divided doses, increased to 4 g in severe infections; CHILD, 30–50 mg/kg daily in divided doses

GENTAMICIN

Indications: septicaemia and neonatal sepsis; meningitis and other CNS infections; biliary tract infection, acute pyelonephritis or prostatitis, endocarditis caused by *Strep. viridans* or *faecalis* (with a penicillin)

Cautions: increase dose interval in renal impairment (see below). Drug interactions: see Appendix 1 (sections 5.1, *5.1, 8, 15*)

Contra-indications: pregnancy, myasthenia gravis

Side-effects: vestibular damage, reversible nephrotoxicity

Dose: by intramuscular injection or slow intravenous injection or infusion, 2–5 mg/kg daily, in divided doses every 8 hours. In renal impairment the interval between successive doses should be increased to 12 hours when the creatinine clearance is 30–70 ml/minute, 24 hours for 10–30 ml/minute, 48 hours for 5–10 ml/minute, and 3–4 days after dialysis for less than 5 ml/minute
CHILD, up to 2 weeks, 3 mg/kg every 12 hours; 2 weeks–12 years, 2 mg/kg every 8 hours

By intrathecal injection, 1 mg daily, with 2–4 mg/kg daily *by intramuscular injection* in divided doses every 8 hours

PHENOXYMETHYLPENICILLIN
(Penicillin V)

Indications: tonsillitis, otitis media, erysipelas, rheumatic fever prophylaxis, endocarditis prophylaxis

Cautions; Contra-indications; Side-effects: see under Benzylpenicillin. Drug interactions: see Appendix 1 (section 5.1)

Dose: 250–500 mg every 6 hours, at least 30 minutes before food; CHILD, every 6 hours, up to 1 year 62.5 mg, 1–5 years 125 mg, 6–12 years 250 mg

TETRACYCLINE

Indications: exacerbations of chronic bronchitis; infections due to brucella, chlamydia, mycoplasma, and rickettsia; severe acne vulgaris

Cautions: breast-feeding; rarely causes photosensitivity. Avoid intravenous administration in hepatic impairment. Drug interactions: see Appendix 1 (sections *2.8C*, 5.1, *7, 9*)

Contra-indications: renal failure, pregnancy, children under 12 years of age

Side-effects: nausea, vomiting, diarrhoea; superinfection with resistant organisms; rarely allergic reactions

Dose: by mouth, 250–500 mg every 6 hours
Acne, see section 13.6
Syphilis, 30–40 g in divided doses over 10–15 days
Non-gonococcal urethritis, 500 mg 4 times daily for 10–21 days

By intramuscular injection, 100 mg every 8–12 hours, or every 4–6 hours in severe infections

By intravenous infusion, 500 mg every 12 hours; max. 2 g daily

3.4   Case history: William Hudson

Task 8   🔲

Study these case notes from Mr Hudson's consultation, part of which you studied in 2.4. Try to work out the meanings of the circled abbreviations. Check your answers in Appendix 2.

The case notes record the doctor's findings on examination. Write down what you would say to Mr Hudson when carrying out this examination.

SURNAME Hudson	**FIRST NAMES** William Henry

AGE   65   **SEX**   M   **MARITAL STATUS**   W

OCCUPATION   Retired postmaster

PRESENT COMPLAINT   Headaches for 4 mths. Wt loss. Headaches feel "like a heavy weight". No nausea or visual symptoms.
No appetite.
Diff. starting to (PU).   Nocturia x3.

O/E
General Condition

ENT

RS   chest clear

CVS   P 110/min irreg.   (? AF)
         BP $\frac{160}{105}$ (HS)   I, II
GIS   (abdo.)   NAD

GUS   (p.r.) prostate moderately enlarged

CNS   (NAD)

IMMEDIATE PAST HISTORY

POINTS OF NOTE
   Wife died (4/12) ago of (Ca.) ovary.

INVESTIGATIONS

Task 9

You decide to refer Mr Hudson for further treatment. The surgeon is Mr Fielding. Write a letter to him outlining Mr Hudson's problems. Use the form below. When you have finished, compare your version with the Key. The case of Mr Hudson continues in 4.4.

Hospital use Only	Clinic	Day Date	Time	Hospital No.	GP112

PARTICULARS OF PATIENT IN BLOCK LETTERS PLEASE

Ambulance Required   Yes / No

Sitting/Stretcher

REQUEST FOR OUT-PATIENT CONSULTATION

Hospital .... Date...................

Urgent Appointment Required   Yes / No

Please arrange for this patient to attend the .... clinic of Dr/Mr ....

Patient's Surname ....   Maiden Surname ....
First Names ....   Single/Married/Widowed/Other
Address ....   Date of Birth ....
Patient's Occupation ....

Postal Code ....   Telephone Number ....
Has the patient attended hospital before YES/NO if "YES" please state:
Name of Hospital ....
Year of Attendance ....   Hospital No...........................
If the patient's name and/or address has/have changed since then please give details:

Name, Address and Telephone Number of
MEDICAL/DENTAL PRACTITIONER

Please use rubber stamp

I would be grateful for your opinion and advice on the above named patient. A brief outline of history, symptoms and signs is given below:

Diagnosis/provisional diagnosis: ....

Present drug treatment and potential special hazards: ....

Relevant X-rays available from: ....   No. (if known) ....

Signature ....

Unit 4   Special examinations

4.1   Instructing, explaining and reassuring

Task 1

Listen to this interview between a hospital consultant, Mr Davidson, and a patient, Mr Priestly. Try to complete the case notes and decide which department the patient has been referred to.

SURNAME		FIRST NAMES	
AGE	SEX	MARITAL STATUS	
OCCUPATION			
PRESENT COMPLAINT			

Task 2

Now listen again to complete the doctor's questions.

1 Can you see any letters at ....(a) ?
2 Well, with the right eye, ...(b) you see ....(c) ?
3 Now does ....(d) make ....(e) difference?
4 What about ....(f) one? Does ....(g) have any effect?

What do you think (d) and (f) refer to?

Task 3

What way would you expect the intonation of these questions to go – up or down? Now listen to the extract again to check your answers.

Language focus 1

Note how the doctor starts the examination:
– *I'd just like to . . .*
– *Could you just . . . for me?*

Note how the doctor indicates the examination is finished:
– *Right, thank you very much indeed.*

Practice 1

You want to examine a patient. Match the examinations in column 1 with the instructions in column 2. Then practise with a partner what you would say to a patient when carrying out these examinations. Rephrase the instructions according to what you have studied in this unit and in Unit 3. For example,

1 (d) I'd just like to examine your throat. Could you just open your mouth as wide as you can?

1	*2*
1 the throat	a) Remove your sock and shoe.
2 the ears	b) Remove your top clothing.
3 the chest	c) Turn your head this way.
4 the back	d) Open your mouth.
5 the foot	e) Tilt your head back.
6 the nasal passage	f) Stand up.

Practice 2

What do you think the doctor is examining for each of these instructions?

1 I want you to push as hard as you can against my hand.
2 Breathe in as far as you can. Now out as far as you can.
3 Say 99. Now whisper it.
4 Could you fix your eyes on the tip of my pen and keep your eyes on it?
5 I want you to keep this under your tongue until I remove it.
6 Would you roll over on your left side and bend your knees up? This may be a bit uncomfortable.
7 I want to see you take your right heel and run it down the front of your left leg.
8 Put out your tongue. Say Aah.

Role-play 1

Work in pairs. **A** should start.

A: Play the part of Mr Davidson.
1   Greet the patient.
2   Indicate that you have had a letter of referral.
3   Ask about the duration of the problem.
4   Ask about his occupation.
5   Ask about the effect on his occupation.
6   Indicate that you would like to examine him.
7   Ask him to read the chart.
8   Ask about the right eye.
9   You change the lens – does it make any difference?
10 You try another one.
11 Indicate that the examination is over.

B: Play the part of Mr Priestly. Use the case notes as prompts.

Task 4

Listen to this extract and tick off the systems examined.

System	Examined
ENT	
RS	
CVS	
GIS	
GUS	
CNS	
Others (specify)	

What kind of examination is this?
How old do you think the patient is?
How do you know?

Language focus 2

Note how the doctor carefully reassures the patient by explaining what she
is going to do and indicating that everything is all right:
– Can I have a look at you *to find out* where your bad cough is coming from?
  ... *That's fine.*

Task 5

Try to complete the doctor's explanations and expressions of reassurance. One word is missing for each blank.
Now listen to the extract again and check your answers.

1 Now I'm ....(a) to put this thing on your chest.
2 It's ....(b) a stethoscope.
3 It ....(c) be a bit cold.
4 OK? First .... (d) all, I listen .... (e) your front and ....(f) your back.
5 Well ....(g), you didn't move at all.
6 Now I'd ....(h) to see your tummy, ...(i) will you lie on the bed for a minute?
7 Now while ....(j) lying there, ...(k) feel your neck and under your arms.
8 Are you ....(l)?
9 ....(m) the top of your legs.
10 That's ....(n). Very quick, ...(o) it?

Listen again. Try to note the intonation of the question forms.

Task 6

Look back to Practice 1. How would you rephrase the instructions for a 4-year-old?

4.2   Rephrasing, encouraging and prompting

Task 7   ▭

The form below is used to measure mental impairment. Discuss with a partner:

1 in what order you might ask these questions;
2 in what form you might ask them.

Listen to the interview between a doctor and a patient he has known for years. Number the questions in the order they are asked. Compare the order with the one you predicted.

ISAACS-WALKEY MENTAL IMPAIRMENT MEASUREMENT

Date of test   /   /

Ask the patient the following questions.
Score 1 for a correct answer, 0 for an error.

		Score
1	What is the name of this place?	....
2	What day of the week is it today?	....
3	What month is it?	....
4	What year is it?	....
5	What age are you? (allow ±1 year error)	....
6	In what year were you born?	....
7	In what month is your birthday?	....
8	What time is it? (allow ±1 hour error)	....
9	How long have you been here? (allow 25% error)	....

Total score   ....

Significance of score

8 or 9	No significant impairment
5 to 7	Moderate impairment
1 to 4	Severe impairment
0	Complete failure

Signature of examiner...

Complete Task 8 before you check your answers in the Key.

Task 8 🔲

Study the information about the patient given below. Then listen to the interview again with the purpose of giving the patient a score.

SURNAME	Walters		**FIRST NAMES**	John Edward	

AGE	83	**SEX**	M	**MARITAL STATUS**	W

OCCUPATION   Retired millworker

PRESENT COMPLAINT

Date of test: Thursday 27 February 1986.
Patient's DOB: 17 April 1902.

How does your score compare with that given by your neighbour and in the Key?

Language focus 3

Note how the doctor uses a rephrasing technique to encourage the patient and give him time to answer. For example,

Question 9: Have you been here long?
              In this house, have you been here long?
              How long have you been living in the High Street?

Note also that the rephrased question is often preceded by an expression like *Do you remember . . .?* For example,
– *Do you remember where this is? Where is this place?*

Task 9 🔲

Predict the missing words in these extracts. Several words are required for most of the extracts. Then listen again to the interview to check your predictions. Try to match the rephrasings with the corresponding test questions. Example (a) is done for you.

a) Question ....**6**...: Do you remember when you were born?
                  What ....(1)?
                  Can you ....(2)?

b) Question ....: Do you remember what time of the month?
                  What ....(3)?

c) Question ....: How old will you be now ....(4)?

d) Question ....: What year is it? Do you ....(5)?   ⟫→

e) Question ....: Fine, and what month are we in?
Well ....(6)?

f) Question ....: Do you remember what day of the week it is?
Or do the ....(7) now that you're
....(8)?

What way would you expect the intonation to go? Listen again and check whether your predictions are correct. Note that the speaker uses falling intonation in questions (a), (b) and (f) because he is expecting more than the answer Yes/No.

Practice 3

Look back at the test form. Think of at least two ways of rephrasing each question.

Task 10

Mr Jameson (see 3.1) was referred to a neurologist for examination. During the examination the neurologist did the following:

a) touched Mr Jameson with a needle;
b) touched Mr Jameson with a piece of cotton wool;
c) touched Mr Jameson with hot and cold tubes;
d) touched Mr Jameson with a vibrating fork.

Listen to the examination and number the steps in the order that the neurologist carried them out.

Language focus 4

Note how the neurologist explained what he was going to do at the first stage of the examination:
– *I now want to ...*
– *I'm going to ...*
– *I'll ...*

Listen to Part 1 of the interview to complete these explanations.
Listen to Parts 2, 3 and 4 and note down:

a) how the doctor explains his intention;
b) how the doctor instructs the patient.

Language focus 5

Note how the doctor marks the sequence of his examinations:
– I *now* want to ...
– *Now* I'm going to ...

Practice 4

Using the prompts from Task 10, try to explain and instruct Mr Jameson through the examination. Remember to use sequence markers.

Practice 5

The neurologist then examined Mr Jameson's leg pulses. The sequence of examination was as follows:

1 the groin;
2 behind the knee;
3 behind the ankle bone;
4 the top of the foot;
5 the other leg.

Try to work out what you would say to Mr Jameson.

Task 11

Listen to Part 5 of the interview and note down:

a) the markers of explanation;
b) the markers of sequence.

Role-play 2

Work in pairs.

Think about other specialist examinations from your own field. Work out what you might explain and instruct the patient. Then find a new partner on whom you can try it out.

4.3 Reading skills: reading articles I

Task 12

Here are headings that are commonly used in articles from American journals. Number them in the order that you would expect them to feature.

References
Report of case
Authors
Introduction
Abstract
Comment
Title

Task 13

Here are some extracts from an article that featured in an American journal – *Archives of Internal Medicine* (January 1985), 145, 140–1. Under what heading, and in what order would you expect to find them?

a)

At present, there are only a few reports on acquired AV fistula of the internal mammary artery. This abnormality is rarely encountered, possibly because the peculiar structure of the bony and cartilaginous thorax offers protection to the blood vessels. These fistulas are of neoplasmic, traumatic, and iatrogenic origin.[1] Several investigators have reported iatrogenic AV fistula of the internal mammary artery after mastectomy,[2] with an indwelling pericardial catheter[3] and after sternotomy.[4,5] In 1982, Keller et al[6] reported a case resembling ours, in which AV fistula was observed between the internal mammary artery and innominate vein after subclavian vein catheterization.

In our case, no symptoms, other than continuous murmur with systolic accentuation, were observed. The patient had chronic renal failure and had undergone treatment with hemodialysis. Consequently, closure of this fistula was considered because of the possible cardiac complications caused by shunt flow from the AV fistula. However, surgical therapy by ligation seemed to be risky in this patient, requiring the postoperative control of renal function. Conventional therapy of transcatheter embolization with small particulate materials may result in pulmonary infarction. To avoid such a risk, transcatheter therapy with stainless-steel coils was chosen. This form of therapy was introduced by Gianturco et al[7] as a relatively easy and effective method, as confirmed by animal and clinical studies in 1975. Since then, it has been widely applied not only for AV fistula, but also for nonsurgical treatment of neoplasm[8] and gastrointestinal tract bleeding.[9]

In our case, the right internal mammary artery was almost completely closed with the stainless-steel coils, however the projection of the coil spring into the right subclavian artery was complicated probably due to unfair technique. Although the possibility of thromboembolic disorder of the distal artery was entertained, no such disorder existed for a relatively long period (six months). For this reason, both thrombocytopenia in chronic renal failure and an anticoagulant regimen for hemodialysis would protect the formation of small thrombi. The angiogram of the right subclavian artery performed in our patient six months later showed no evidence of stenosis of the artery, as well as the complete closure of the AV fistula.

b)

● **We encountered a case of right internal mammary artery to innominate vein fistula following subclavian vein catheterization and the projection of the coil spring was projected after transcatheter intravascular coil occlusion. We were worried about both distal thromboembolism from small thrombi forming on a portion of the coil spring and stenosis of the subclavian artery. However, there was no evidence of thromboembolism of the distal artery, and good patency of the right subclavian artery was shown by an angiogram performed six months later. The patient has been receiving heparin therapy during hemodialysis, which should help prevent thromboembolism of the distal artery.**
(***Arch Intern Med*** 1985; 145: 140–141)

c)

Although acquired arteriovenous (AV) fistula of the internal mammary artery is rarely observed,[1–6] to our knowledge, there have been no reports on the projection of the proximal coil spring into another artery after transcatheter intravascular coil occlusion.

We saw a case of iatrogenic AV fistula complicated by the projection of the coil spring after occlusion by the transcatheter intravascular method. The long-term findings are reported.

d)

1. Senno A, Schweitzer P, Merrill C, et al: Arteriovenous fistulas of the internal mammary artery: Review of the literature. *J Cardiovasc Surg* 1975; 16:296–301.

2. Glenn F, Steinberg I: Arteriovenous fistula of the right internal mammary vessels following radical mastectomy: Visualization by angiocardiography. *J Thorac Surg* 1957;33:719–722.

3. Silverstein R, Crumbo D, Long DL, et al: Iatrogenic arteriovenous fistula: An unusual complication of indwelling pericardial catheter and intrapericardial steroid instillation for the treatment of uremic pericarditis. *Arch Intern Med* 1978; 138:308–310.

4. Longmaid HE, Jay M, Phillips D: Angiographic evaluation of post-sternotomy arteriovenous fistula of the internal mammary artery and vein. *Cardiovasc Intervent Radiol* 1980;3:150–152.

5. Maher TD, Glenn JF, Magovern GJ: Internal mammary arteriovenous fistula after sternotomy. *Arch Surg* 1982;117:1100–1101.

6. Keller FS, Rösch J, Banner RL, et al: Iatrogenic internal mammary artery-to-innominate vein fistula: Percutaneous nonsurgical closure. *Chest* 1982;81: 255–257.

7. Gianturco C, Anderson JH, Wallace S: Mechanical devices for arterial occlusion. *AJR* 1975; 124:428–435.

8. Layne TA, Finck EJ, Boswell WD: Transcatheter occlusion of the arterial supply to arteriovenous fistulas with Gianturco coils. *AJR* 1978; 131:1027–1030.

9. Clark RA, Frey RT, Colley DP, et al: Transcatheter embolization of hepatic arteriovenous fistulas for control of hemobilia. *Gastrointest Radiol* 1981; 6:353–356.

e)

Tsugihiro Nakamura, MD; Yasuhide Nakashima, MD; Kogi Yu, MD; Yatuka Senda, MD; Osamu Hasegawa, MD; Akio Kuroiwa, MD; Yoshiki Tsukamoto, MD

f)

To insert a central vein pressure catheter for fluid control, puncture of the right subclavian vein using the right infraclavicular approach was tried several times immediately after hospital admission. Uremia was controlled by peritoneal dialysis and hemodialysis; no further disturbance of consciousness was observed. On the second hospital day, however, continuous machinery murmur was auscultated in the right clavicular area; phonocardiography revealed high-pitched continuous murmur with systolic accentuation (Fig 1, left). An AV fistula between the right internal mammary artery and the innominate vein with false aneurysm was assumed by selective right subclavian arteriography (Fig 2, top); iatrogenic AV fistula was diagnosed. The transcatheter intravascular coil occlusion was conducted because of the patient's relatively higher surgical risk and history of chronic renal failure. Right subclavian arteriography after the occlusion of the AV fistula indicated that the fistula was almost closed. It showed, however, that the proximal coil spring was projecting into the right subclavian artery (Fig 2, center). Because of this finding, we were worried about the possibility of thromboembolism of distal artery. However, the patient had no evidence of thromboembolism for six months. The patient was reexamined by right subclavian arteriography six months later. There was no pathologic stenosis of the subclavian artery, and complete closure of the AV fistula (Fig 2, bottom). No continuous murmur was found by phonocardiography at that time (Fig 1, right).

g)

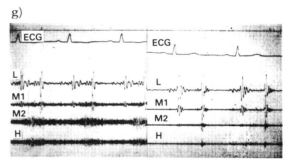

Fig. 1. – Phonocardiograms recorded on first intercostal space of right sternal border before (left) and after (right) transcatheter intravascular coil occlusion. Left, High-pitched continuous murmur with systolic accentuation. Right, No continuous murmur. L indicates magnitude of frequencies below 50 Hz attenuated (6 dB/octave); M1, magnitude of frequencies below 100 Hz attenuated (12 dB/octave); M2, magnitude of frequencies below 200 Hz attenuated (24 dB/octave); and H, magnitude of frequencies below 400 Hz attenuated (24 dB/octave).

Task 14

Now read the article again carefully. Three parts of the article are missing. Can you identify them and make any suggestions as to their nature?

Task 15

Here is one of the missing parts. Try to complete it by filling each space with one word.

A 20-year-old woman .... (1) admitted .... (2) the hospital of the University of Occupational and Environmental Health, Japan, ... (3) of edema and disturbance of consciousness due .... (4) uremia. .... (5) patient .... (6) been receiving peritoneal dialysis .... (7) another hospital because .... (8) high levels .... (9) blood urea nitrogen (194 mg/dl) and nausea, vomiting, and edema following .... (10) symptoms of .... (11) common cold. The patient .... (12) a history .... (13) proteinuria .... (14) childhood and .... (15) hypertension one year prior .... (16) being seen.

The patient .... (17) in a comatose state .... (18) admission .... (19) the hospital. Her BP .... (20) 60/30 mm Hg and her pulse rate .... (21) 88 beats per minute. She .... (22) anemia, ... (23) no jaundice. Heart sounds .... (24) normal. A 3/6 ejection systolic murmur and moist rales .... (25) auscultated .... (26) the left sternal border and .... (27) the lung region, respectively. Edema .... (28) observed .... (29) the lower extremities. Azotemia and serious anemia .... (30) also noted.

Note the American spellings 'edema' and 'anemia'.

4.4   Case history: William Hudson

Task 16

Mr Hudson was put on a waiting list for a TUR following his consultation with Mr Fielding. However, after five weeks he was admitted to hospital as an emergency. Study the registrar's case notes on Mr Hudson following his admission.

PRESENT COMPLAINT
Unable to PU for 24hrs.
In severe pain.
Awaiting TUR for enlarged prostate.

O/E
General Condition   Restlessness due to pain.
                          Sweating ++.

ENT

RS   Chest clear.

CVS   P 120   AF
              BP $\frac{180}{120}$ HS I, II no murmurs.

GIS

                          bladder distended to
                          umbilicus
GUS
              PR prostate enlarged, soft.

CNS   NAD

DIAGNOSIS
(1) Acute retention due to prostate hypertrophy.
(2) Atrial fibrillation   ? cause.

MANAGEMENT
Sedate
Catheterise
Ask physician to see him

The following notes were added after catheterisation:

INVESTIGATIONS
urinalysis   3+ sugar

MANAGEMENT

R_x digoxin   0.25 mg daily
        metformin   500 mg t.d.s.

What addition would you make to the Diagnosis section?
Write a letter to Mr Hudson's doctor, Dr Watson, explaining your findings.

Unit 5   Investigations

5.1   Explaining and discussing investigations

Task 1

In this extract a hospital doctor prepares a patient for a lumbar puncture. The patient has been ill for a week with headaches and a temperature following a respiratory infection. Examination shows neck stiffness. During the extract the doctor instructs the patient to take up the correct position for the lumbar puncture. Try to predict his instructions from these clues. Each blank may represent one or several missing words.

1 Now I want you to move right to the edge of the bed.
2 Lie on ....
3 Now can you bend both your ....?
4 Put your head ....
5 Curl ....
6 Lie ....

Task 2

Listen to the extract and check your predictions.

Language focus 1

In the extract above the doctor tries to do three things:

1 Explain what he is going to do and why.
   Now I'm going to take some fluid off your back *to find out* what's giving you these headaches.
2 Instruct the patient to take up the correct position.
   Now I want you to move right to the edge of the bed.
3 Reassure the patient about the investigation.
   It won't take very long.
   Now I'm going to give you a local anaesthetic *so it won't be sore.*

Practice 1

Here is part of a doctor's explanation during a sternal marrow. The explanation (opposite) has been put in the wrong order. Try to rearrange it.

52

a) Now I'm going to give you an injection of local anaesthetic. First into the skin and then into the bone.
b) Then we'll put a dressing over the area.
c) Now the next thing I'm going to do is to put a towel, a clean towel, over the area.
d) First of all, I'm just going to wash the area with a bit of antiseptic.
e) Just going to remove the needle from your chest.
f) Now we're ready to do the actual test.
g) Now I'm going to remove the actual cells from your bone.

Language focus 2

Doctors often combine reassurance with a warning. Study these examples from a sternal marrow investigation:
– It shouldn't be painful, *but you will be aware of a feeling of pressure.*
– *This may feel a little bit uncomfortable,* but it won't take long.

Practice 2

Practise with a fellow student preparing a patient for the following investigations. Explain, instruct, reassure and warn where necessary.

1 ECG / man, 68 / ? myocardial infarction
2 barium meal / woman, 23 / ? duodenal ulcer
3 Crosby capsule / girl, 6 / ? coeliac disease
4 ultrasound scan / woman, 26 / baby small for dates at 32 weeks
5 myelogram / man, 53 / carpenter / ? prolapsed intervertebral disc

Task 3

Study this list of investigations for a 43-year-old salesman who presents with a blood pressure of 200 over 130. Then list them into the three categories below. Add any others you consider essential.

ECG   barium meal
serum cholesterol   creatinine
IVP (IVU)   skull X-ray
serum thyroxine   radioisotope studies
chest X-ray   urea and electrolytes
urinalysis   uric acid

Essential	Possibly useful	Not required

Now listen to three doctors discussing this case and the investigations. Note how they group the investigations. Have you grouped them in the same way?

Language focus 3

Note these expressions used *between doctors* in discussing a choice of investigations.

Essential	Possibly useful	Not required

should
must
be + required
    essential
    important
    indicated
	could	need not
		
		be + not necessary
		    required
		    important

Essential not to do		
should not must not be + contraindicated		

For example,
– The patient *should* be given an X-ray.
– *It is important* to give an X-ray.
– An X-ray *is indicated* (formal).

Practice 3

Study these brief case notes and choose only the most appropriate investigations from the list which follows each case. Add any other investigations you think essential. Then work in pairs. Take three cases each. Explain to each other your choice of investigations for these patients. If you are working alone, write down your explanation.

a)

SURNAME Gumley	FIRST NAMES John

AGE 60	SEX M	MARITAL STATUS M

OCCUPATION   Electrician

PRESENT COMPLAINT
  Coughing up blood. Has temp. Smoker.

O/E
General Condition   finger clubbing, air entry ↓ L mid zone

chest X-ray   sputum culture
bronchoscopy   serum proteins
urinalysis

b)

SURNAME	Sharp	FIRST NAMES	Emma

AGE 43	SEX	F	MARITAL STATUS	M

OCCUPATION   Housewife

PRESENT COMPLAINT

abdominal pain, heavy periods

O/E
General Condition

abdominal ultrasonograph   chest X-ray
Hb   LFTS
EUA and D & C

c)

SURNAME	Donaldson	FIRST NAMES	Grace

AGE 23	SEX F	MARITAL STATUS	S

OCCUPATION   Schoolteacher

PRESENT COMPLAINT

agitation, difficulty in sleeping, ↑ appetite
↓ wt

O/E
General Condition   warm, sweaty skin, tachycardia, soft goitre
                        with bruit

angiogram   serum thyroxine
CAT scan of skull T_3 resin uptake ratio

⟫→

d)

SURNAME Pritt	FIRST NAMES William
AGE 44 **SEX** M	**MARITAL STATUS** D
OCCUPATION Printer	
PRESENT COMPLAINT abdominal pain after eating fatty foods	
O/E **General Condition** obese ++, tender R hypochondrium	

cholecystogram   ECG
MSU   endoscopy
barium meal   abdominal ultrasonograph

e)

SURNAME Scott	FIRST NAMES Barry
AGE 2½ **SEX** M	**MARITAL STATUS**
OCCUPATION —	
PRESENT COMPLAINT sore throat, mother says he has a temp. and rash	
O/E **General Condition** occipital glands enlarged and tender, maculopapular rash behind ears and spreading down trunk	

chest X-ray   monospot
throat swab   viral antibodies
serum iron   full blood count

f)

SURNAME Lock	FIRST NAMES Mary
AGE 68 **SEX** F	**MARITAL STATUS** Sep
OCCUPATION Retired waitress	
PRESENT COMPLAINT dull ache above R eye, sees haloes round lights	
O/E **General Condition** hazy cornea, pupil half - dilated and fixed	

tonometry   skull X-ray
swab from cornea to bacteriology

Role-play 1

Work in pairs. **B** should start.

A: Play the part of the patient for one of the six cases above. In case (e) you are a parent. You want to know why the investigations are required, what the investigations involve, and if the investigations will be painful.
B: Play the part of the doctor. Explain the investigations required and answer any questions raised.

5.2 Using medical documents

Task 4

Listen to this telephone call from a haematology lab to a doctor's surgery. As you listen, record the results of the investigations in the correct spaces on the form below. The patient is Mr Kevin Hall (see 1.1 and 1.2).

```
┌─────────────────────────────────────────────────┐
│           TELEPHONE REPORT FROM                  │
│         HAEMATOLOGY LABORATORY                    │
│                                                   │
│  PATIENTS NAME          UNIT NO                    │
│                                                   │
│  ...............................................  │
│  ───────────────────────────────                  │
│                                                   │
│                         BLOOD FILM                │
│                                                   │
│  WBC x10⁹/L ............  NEUTRO .......... %      │
│                                                   │
│  Hb g/dl ...............  LYMPH .......... %       │
│                                                   │
│  Hct ...................  MONO ........... %       │
│                                                   │
│  MCVfl .................  EOSINO ......... %       │
│                                                   │
│  Platelets x10⁹/L ......  BASO ........... %       │
│                                                   │
│  ESR mm ................                           │
│                                                   │
│                                                   │
│            OTHER INFORMATION                      │
│                                                   │
│  ...............................................  │
│  ...............................................  │
│  ...............................................  │
│                                                   │
│  PROTHROMBIN RATIO ..................... :1        │
│                                                   │
│  TIME MESSAGE RECEIVED ........... AM/PM           │
│                                                   │
│  MESSAGE RECEIVED BY ...................           │
│                                                   │
│  DATE RECEIVED .........................           │
└─────────────────────────────────────────────────┘
```

WBC $\times 10^9$/L .... NEUTRO ...... %

Hb g/dl ...... LYMPH ...... %

Hct ...... MONO ...... %

MCVfl ...... EOSINO ...... %

Platelets $\times 10^9$/L ...... BASO ...... %

ESR mm ......

Task 5

Study the clinical chemistry results for Mr Hall which are shown on the form below. In addition to these results, the patient's urine showed: albumen ++, and a trace of glucose.

```
        DEPARTMENT OF CLINICAL CHEMISTRY

                               GP 5487       HALL    M
        General Hospital       DR. WATSON    GP 01

                      Date  25.05.84
                      Time  00:00
                      Spec  746273
                      No.   746284


        Plasma   SODIUM
          (135-145) mmol/l      158
        PL POTASSIUM
          (3.5-5)    mmol/l     6.2
        Plasma CHLORIDE
          (95-105)   mmol/l     96
        Plasma CO2
          (21-26)    mmol/l     16
        Plasma UREA
          (3.3-6.6) mmol/l      50.1
        PL TOT PROTEIN
          (60-80)    s/l        71
        PL CREATININE
          (.07-.11) mmol/l      0.09
        Plasma GLUCOSE
          (3.9-5.0)             5.1


        Report printed on 30 May 84  3.28 PM
```

Identify which of these results are outside the normal range and describe each of the significant results. These words may be useful:

low	high	abnormal
reduced	raised	
	elevated	

For example,
– *Blood urea is abnormally high.*

Task 6

Kevin Hall's GP phones the hospital to arrange for his admission. Fill in the gaps in his call (see opposite) using the information from the haematology lab, the clinical chemistry results, and the information given in Task 5. Add your own diagnosis.

D: I'm phoning about a 32-year-old man. I saw him a year ago when he
.........................(1) of headaches which had been troubling him for three months. On
examination he was ....(2) to have a blood pressure of 180 over 120.
Urinalysis was ....(3), ECG and chest X-rays were also normal. He was
commenced on a beta ....(4) and ....(5) but his blood pressure
remained slightly ....(6).

On a recent visit he complained of nausea, vomiting and headaches. His blood
pressure was 160 over 120, urinalysis showed ....(7) plus plus and a trace
of glucose. I've just received his lab results. His haemoglobin is ....(8),
ESR ....(9). Blood film showed poikilocytosis plus and ....(10)
cells plus plus. Blood urea was ....(11) raised, ...(12), sodium
158, potassium 6.2, bicarbonate ....(13).

I'd like to arrange his urgent admission for investigation and treatment of
.........................(14).

Task 7

Look back at the case of Peter Green in 1.2. Re-read his case notes and the letter from his GP. List the investigations you would carry out on this patient. Then study these haematological, clinical chemistry and ECG (V5 only) results for Mr Green. Write to his GP, Dr Jones, and describe your findings.

G.P.		
PLEASE PHONE RESULTS	Tick ✓ Appropriate Green Blocks	
URGENT SPECIMEN		
O32	DATE CODE	
462	TEST No.	
O7.1	WBC ×10⁹/l	
4·69	RBC ×10¹²/l	
14.8	Hb g/dl ✓	
.431	Hct	
100·	MCV fl	
34·1	MCH pg	
33.8	MCHC g/dl	
264	PLATELETS ×10⁹/l	
	ESR mm in 1st hour	
RETICULOCYTE ×10⁹/l		
%		
BLOOD FILM		
NEUTROPHILS ×10⁶/l		
%		
LYMPHOCYTES ×10⁶/l		
%		
MONOCYTES ×10⁶/l		
%		
EOSINOPHILS ×10⁶/l		
%		
BASOPHILS ×10⁶/l		
%		

SURNAME: Green
FORENAME: Peter
ADDRESS: 14 Grizzle Lane, Applecross
CONSULTANT/G.P.: Dr Scott
CLINICAL DETAILS
UNIT NUMBER
AGE: 42
SEX: M
WARD/UNIT
G.P.'s ADDRESS: Dr Jones, Health Centre, Applecross
PRIVATE PATIENT — PLEASE INDICATE □
Date Collected / Time / Signature

(LAB USE ONLY) BLOOD FILM WITHIN NORMAL LIMITS □

Normochromic	✓	Normocytic	+ + ✓
Hypochromic		Microcytic	
Polycromasia		Macrocytic	+
Poikilocytosis		Ovalocytes	+

FOR NORMAL VALUES SEE BACK OF THIS SHEET

Sig
DATE OF REPORT: 7/ 10/85
LAB. REF. No.: 462

```
                DEPARTMENT OF CLINICAL CHEMISTRY

Applecross Infirmary            GP 1563526      GREEN    M
                                DR. SCOTT


Date  07/10/85
Time  00:00
Spec  35931
No.   35998



Plasma   SODIUM
  (135-145)  mmol/l      137
Pl  POTASSIUM
  (3.5-5)    mmol/l      4.6
Plasma  CHLORIDE
  (95-105)   mmol/l      96
Plasma  CO2
  (21-26)    mmol/l      22
Plasma  UREA
  (3.3-6.6)  mmol/l      3.6
Pl TOT PROTEIN
  (60-80)    g/l         71
Pl CHOLESTEROL
  (3.9-6.2)  mmol/l      7.2
Pl TOT GLYCEROL
  (0.8-2.1)  mmol/l      1.9


Report printed on 07 – October – 85    4.13 PM
```

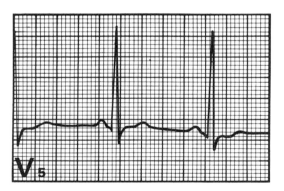

Before exercise

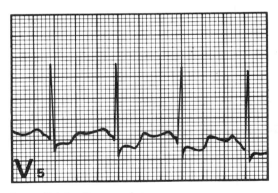

Immediately after exercise

5.3 Reading skills: reading articles II

Task 8

Here are headings that are commonly used in articles from British journals and others that are prepared in accordance with the Vancouver style (International Committee of Medical Journal Editors – 'Uniform requirements for manuscripts submitted to bio-medical journals', *British Medical Journal* (1982) 284, 1766–70). Number them in the order that you would expect them to feature.

Results
Abstract
Discussion
Patients and methods
References
Acknowledgements
Introduction
Authors
Title

Task 9

Here is an extract from an article by J.W.Howie, 'How I read', *British Medical Journal* (1976), 3, 1113–25. How does the procedure he describes compare with your own?

> Keeping up to date is a responsibility in which doctors often fail their patients. Of course, doctors are busy, but they are bad doctors if they stop reading about their subject. Writers must make their articles readable if they are to be read; and they must realise the competitive nature of their quest for readers. During my active professional life I necessarily read a great deal – at home, in trains and buses, in the laboratory and office; but I never read as much as the applicants for posts claimed that they did. Latterly, I read two weekly journals and two periodicals (I had better not say which) besides many manuscripts, reports, contents lists, abstracts, and reprints. I had to be highly selective, and I proceeded as described in this paper through title, summary, results, discussion, introduction, and review of the literature to methods and material in that order. If it helps writers of papers to have this account of one reader's approach I have reached my objective.

⟫→

Here are some extracts from an article in the *British Medical Journal* that illustrate another procedure commonly followed by medical researchers. Work out the procedure by identifying the extracts.

a)

Comparison of barium swallow and ultrasound in diagnosis of gastro-oesophageal reflux in children

b)

Fifty one infants and older children with suspected gastro-oesophageal reflux entered a study comparing the diagnostic accuracy of a standard barium swallow examination with that of ultrasound scanning. All children were examined by both techniques.

In 40 cases there was unequivocal agreement between the examinations. Of the remaining patients, four had definite reflux by ultrasonic criteria but showed no evidence of reflux on barium swallow examination, four had positive findings on ultrasound but showed only minimal reflux on barium swallow, and one showed minimal reflux on ultrasound but had a negative barium meal result. In two children the ultrasound study was inconclusive.

Ultrasound has an important role in the diagnosis and follow up of patients under the age of 5 years with gastro-oesophageal reflux.

c)

Both ultrasound and barium swallow examinations have an important part to play in patients with symptomatic gastro-oesophageal reflux. Barium examinations are useful in the diagnosis of complications of reflux and in detecting uncommon conditions. We emphasise that most children do not require barium meal examination for diagnosis or during the subsequent management of reflux.

d)

Results of barium swallow and ultrasound examinations

	Barium swallow result			
Ultrasonic appearance	Positive	Negative	Minimal positive	Total
Positive	15	4	4	23
Negative		24		24
Minimal positive		1	1	2
Inconclusive	2			2
Total	17	29	5	51

e)

Gastro-oesophageal reflux is an important and relatively common condition in infancy and childhood. It may be physiological, particularly in the younger age group,[1] and is self limiting and benign in most cases.[2] It may, however, be one of the causes of failure to thrive, be a cause of repeated chest infections from aspiration, and be a factor in cot deaths.[3] In addition to radiological means, 24 hour intraluminal oesophageal pH probe monitoring and isotope scintigraphy have been used for detecting gastro-oesophageal reflux. Recently a method using ultrasound has been described.[4]

We report a study comparing the established method of barium swallow examination with ultrasound scanning in children with suspected gastro-oesophageal reflux.

f)

D R NAIK, A BOLIA, D J MOORE

g)

References

1 Carre IJ. Clinical significance of gastro-oesophageal reflux. *Arch Dis Child* 1984; **59**: 911–2.
2 Silverman A, Roy CC. *Pediatric clinical gastroenterology.* 2nd ed. St Louis: C V Mosby, 1983: 10–1.
3 MacFadyne UM, Hendry GMA, Simpson H. Gastro-oesophageal reflux in near-miss sudden infant death syndrome and suspected recurrent aspiration. *Arch Dis Child* 1983; **58**: 87–91.
4 Naik DR, Moore DJ. Ultrasound diagnosis of gastro-oesophageal reflux. *Arch Dis Child* 1984; **59**: 366–7.
5 Levick RK. In: Whitehouse GH, Worthington BS, eds. *Techniques in diagnostic radiology.* London: Blackwell Scientific Publications, 1983: 325–35.
6 Herbst JJ. Gastroesophageal reflux. *J Pediatr* 1981; **98**: 859–70.
7 Fowkes FGR. Containing the use of diagnostic tests. *Br Med J* 1985; **290**: 488–9.

If you were interested in more details of the experiment, what part would you read next?

Task 10

Here is the part that the researcher chose to read next. Try to complete the following using one word for each space.

Fifty one children .... (1) examined .... (2) suspected gastro-oesophageal reflux. .... (3) ages ranged .... (4) 4 days .... (5) 16 years, ... (6) most were under the age .... (7) 5 years. .... (8) main indications .... (9) investigation were vomiting, failure .... (10) thrive, repeated chest infections, ... (11) near miss infant death syndrome. The examinations .... (12) carried .... (13) by two operators independently. One operator carried .... (14) the barium swallow examination, ... (15) was followed later .... (16) the ultrasound examination, carried .... (17) by the second operator .... (18) had no knowledge .... (19) the results .... (20) the barium examination. The technique .... (21) the ultrasound .... (22) detailed elsewhere.[4] Barium swallow examinations .... (23) carried .... (24) using the standard technique.[5]

5.4   Case history: William Hudson

Task 11

Mr Hudson has a transurethral resection of his prostate. His diabetes was controlled by diet and oral hypoglycaemic drugs. He continued with digoxin. The diuretic was discontinued. Four months later he complained of diarrhoea and sickness over a period of two days. He was treated for this, but four days later a neighbour called Mr Hudson's doctor as an emergency. The doctor arranged an immediate admission and wrote a letter to the hospital consultant to accompany Mr Hudson to hospital. Complete the gaps in this letter with the help of the GP's case notes given below.

PRESENT COMPLAINT
Diarrhoea and vomiting for 6 days.

O/E
General Condition   dehydrated and semi - comatose

ENT   NAD

RS   NAD

CVS   P irreg. 110/min   BP $\frac{110}{60}$

GIS   Sl. distension of abdo. No tenderness.
Bowel sounds absent.

GUS   NAD

CNS   Difficulty to arouse. Responds to painful stimuli.

IMMEDIATE PAST HISTORY
Diabetic on metformin 500 mg t.d.s
and digoxin 0.25 mg for CCF. TUR 4/12 ago.

POINTS OF NOTE

INVESTIGATIONS

DIAGNOSIS
? diabetic coma following acute gastro - enteritis

Dear Mr Fielding,

Thank you for arranging to admit Mr Hudson. He is a 66-year-old widower
who has had .... (1) and vomiting for six days. He is
a diabetic on .... (2) , 500mg, ... (3)
times daily and also takes digoxin for mild .... (4)
failure. When our nurse visited him four days ago, his general condition
was good but when I called to see him today, I found him
.... (5) and .... (6) . He still has
diarrhoea although vomiting has stopped. He is apyrexial, blood pressure
is 110/60 and his pulse weak and .... (7) at 110 per
minute. The .... (8) is slightly distended although
there is no .... (9) . Bowel sounds are
.... (10) .

Diagnosis: ? acute gastroenteritis leading to .... (11)
diabetic coma. By the way, he had a .... (12) four
months ago which was uncomplicated.

Yours sincerely,

Dr Peter Watson

Role-play 2

Work in pairs. **B** should start.

A: Play the part of the consultant. Explain briefly the investigations you intend
to carry out on Mr Hudson and his present condition.
B: Play the part of Mr Hudson's son or daughter. You are concerned about
your father. Find out what is wrong with him and ask what the consultant
is going to do to help your father.

Unit 6 Making a diagnosis

6.1 Discussing a diagnosis

Task 1 ▱

Listen to this extract in which a doctor interviews a 59-year-old office worker.
As you listen, note the patient's present complaint.

SURNAME Nicol		FIRST NAMES Harvey
AGE 59	SEX M	MARITAL STATUS M
OCCUPATION Office worker		
PRESENT COMPLAINT		
O/E General Condition ENT RS		

Complete Tasks 2, 3 and 4 before you check your answers in the Key.

Task 2 ▱

Listen to the extract again and write down several possible diagnoses for this
patient. You will be given further information on him later.

1 ....

2 ....

3 ....

4 ....

5 ....

Complete Tasks 3 and 4 before you check your answers in the Key.

Task 3

Here are the doctor's findings on examination.

O/E				
General Condition	Good	T	37.4°	
ENT				
RS				
CVS	P 80/min reg.		BP 160/95	
	HS normal		left temporal artery palpable	
GIS				
GUS				
CNS	No neck stiffness. Fundi normal.			
	Neck movts full with no pain.			

Look back at the possible diagnoses you listed in Task 2. Order them so that the most likely diagnosis is first and the least likely last. Exclude any which now seem very unlikely.

1 ....

2 ....

3 ....

4 ....

5 ....

Which investigations would you check for this patient? Write them here.

INVESTIGATIONS

Complete Task 4 before you check your answers in the Key.

Task 4

The results of some investigations for this patient are given on page 102. How do these findings affect your diagnosis? Write your final diagnosis here.

```
DIAGNOSIS



```

Language focus 1

Note these expressions used *between doctors* in discussing a diagnosis.

	Certain	*Fairly certain*	*Uncertain*
Yes	is must	seems probably likely	might could may
No	can't definitely not exclude rule out	unlikely	possibly a possibility

After the listening extract we have little information on which to base our diagnosis. We are still uncertain. We can say:
– The patient *might* have cervical spondylosis.
– Cervical spondylosis is a *possibility*.

Discuss your other diagnoses in Task 2 in the same way.
The findings on examination provide more evidence for a diagnosis. Some diagnoses become more likely while others become less likely. We can say:
– He *seems* to have temporal arteritis.
– There is no neck stiffness. It's *unlikely* that he's got cervical spondylosis.

Discuss the diagnoses you listed in Task 3 in the same way.
The results of the investigations provide stronger evidence for our final diagnosis. We can say:
– A raised ESR makes temporal arteritis *very likely*.
– Normal skull X-ray *excludes* a space-occupying lesion.
– He *can't* have a space-occupying lesion.

Finally, following the biopsy, we can say:
– He *must* have temporal arteritis.

Practice 1

In this exercise, try to make a diagnosis on the basis of the information given on each patient. The exercise is in three stages. At each stage you are given more information to help you make a final diagnosis. Discuss your diagnoses at each stage.

STAGE A

1 The patient is a 26-year-old woman complaining of swelling of the ankles.
2 The patient is a 5-year-old girl with a petechial rash.
3 The patient is a 28-year-old man with headaches, sore throat and enlarged glands in the neck.
4 The patient is a 40-year-old woman complaining of nausea and episodes of pain in the right hypochondrium.
5 The patient is a 49-year-old man exhibiting Raynaud's phenomenon and with difficulty in swallowing.

Do not look ahead until you have considered a diagnosis for each patient.

STAGE B

1 Pregnancy test is negative. Chest X-ray is normal. Pulse is normal. The liver is not enlarged.
2 Both ankles, the left elbow and the right wrist are swollen and painful. The history shows no ingestion of drugs. Bone marrow is normal.
3 The spleen is palpable and there is a macropapular rash all over.
4 The pain is associated with dietary indiscretion. Murphy's sign is positive. There is mild jaundice.
5 The patient exhibits cutaneous calcinosis and has difficulty in breathing.

Do not look ahead until you have considered a diagnosis for each patient.

STAGE C

1 Five day fecal fat collection is 15 mmol/l. Jejunal biopsy is normal. Lab stick urinary protein test shows protein + +. Serum total protein is 40 g/l.
2 The rash is on the buttocks and extensor surfaces of the arms and legs.
3 WBC shows lymphocytes + +. Monospot is positive.
4 Lab tests show alkaline phosphotase 160 units/l. Cholecystography shows a non-functioning gall bladder.
5 The patient's face is pinched.

6.2   Explaining a diagnosis

Task 5

Look back at Task 1 in Unit 3. In that extract a doctor was examining a patient suffering from leg and back pain. An X-ray of the lumbar spine confirmed that the patient had a prolapsed intervertebral disc. Think about how you would explain this diagnosis to the patient. Write down the points you would include in your explanation. List the points in the best order. For example,

1 how serious the problem is

Task 6   🔲

In this extract the doctor is explaining the diagnosis to the patient. As you listen, note the points covered and the order in which they are dealt with. Then compare your own list in Task 5 with the list you have noted.

Language focus 2   🔲

When explaining a diagnosis, a patient would expect you to answer the following questions:

1 What's the cause of my problem?
2 How serious is it?
3 What are you going to do about it?
4 What are the chances of a full recovery?

In Unit 7, we will deal with questions 3 and 4. Here we will look at some of the language used to answer questions 1 and 2.
In explanations it is important to use straightforward, non-specialist language with only such detail as is important for the patient's understanding of the problem. The language of the textbooks you may have studied is clearly unsuitable for patient explanation. Compare this extract with the recorded explanation above.

Herniation of part of a lumbar intervertebral disc is a common cause of combined back pain and sciatica . . . Part of the gelatinous nucleus pulposus protrudes through a rent in the annulus fibrosus at its weakest part, which is postero-lateral . . . If it is large, the protrusion herniates through the posterior ligament and may impinge upon an issuing nerve to cause sciatic pain.

(J. C. Adams, *Outline of Orthopaedics*, 10th ed. (Edinburgh: Churchill Livingstone, 1986), p. 217).

You can make sure your explanations are easily understood by avoiding medical terminology where possible and defining the terms you use in a simple way. Note how the doctor describes a disc: . . . *The disc is a little pad of gristle which lies between the bones in your spine.*

Practice 2

Try to describe these terms in a simple way for a patient to understand.

1 the pancreas   5 arrhythmia
2 the thyroid   6 bone marrow
3 fibroids   7 the prostate gland
4 emphysema   8 gastro-oesophageal reflux

Language focus 3

Explanations often involve describing causes and effects. Look at these examples:

cause	*effect*
bend the knee	the tension is taken off the nerve
straighten it	the nerve goes taut

We can link a cause and an effect like this:
— *If we bend the knee, the tension is taken off the nerve.*
— *If we straighten it, the nerve goes taut.*

Note that both the cause and effect are in the present tense because we are describing something which is generally true.

Practice 3

Write a suitable effect for each of these causes. Then link each cause and effect pair to make a simple statement you could use in an explanation to a patient. Indicate the problem you are trying to explain to the patient. For example,

cause	*effect*
You lift a heavy load without bending your knees.	You may damage a disc in your spine.

— *If you lift a heavy load without bending your knees, you may damage a disc in your spine.*

Problem: prolapsed intervertebral disc

1 The stomach produces too much acid.
2 A woman gets German measles during pregnancy.
3 You vomit several times in quick succession.
4 Your skin is in contact with certain plants.
5 Your blood pressure remains high.
6 You give your baby too much fruit.
7 The cholesterol level in the blood gets too high.
8 There are repeated injuries to a joint.

Role-play 1

Work in pairs. **A** should start.

A: Play the part of a doctor. Explain these diagnoses to the following patients.
1 Hypertension: 50-year-old man, director of a small company.
2 Insulin-dependent diabetes: 11-year-old girl accompanied by her mother.
3 Osteoarthritis of the left hip: 65-year-old retired schoolteacher.
4 Epilepsy: 23-year-old lorry driver.
5 Carcinoma of the bowel: 52-year-old cook.
6 A depressive illness: 27-year-old teacher of handicapped children.
7 Atopic eczema: 6-month-old baby boy accompanied by his mother.

B: Play the part of the patients. In 2 and 7, play the part of a parent.

6.3   Reading skills: reading articles III

Task 7

Here are some extracts from an article in the *British Medical Journal* given in the order that they were read. Try to identify them to work out the procedure used and suggest a suitable title.

a)
The practice of preoperative assessment in 24 departments of anaesthesia in Great Britain and Ireland was surveyed. Most departments had no rigid policies governing assessment, and many served several hospitals. There was little evidence that admission procedures of patients scheduled for surgery or the organisation of operating lists took account of the problems encountered by anaesthetists undertaking preoperative assessment.

From the participating departments 415 anaesthetists completed a questionnaire of their individual practice. Most (57%) visited at least 80% of their patients preoperatively, but 22% saw less than 50% of patients. The detection of potential anaesthetic problems and the establishment of rapport with patients were highly rated reasons for conducting such visits. Failure to visit was often related to organisational defects within the hospital service, and anaesthetists saw little prospect of improving these defects. The demands created by the needs of preoperative assessment on the one hand, and the need for a rapid turnover of surgical patients and financial stringency on the other, conflict, and this conflict is not easily reconciled.

b)
There have been public expressions in the press of disquiet regarding the lack of preoperative assessment; patients may understandably prefer to meet their anaesthetist, though this study did not seek to explore this. Besides the press, society as a whole expresses its will through the courts. The defence organisations have settled claims on behalf of surgeons when failure to conduct preoperative assessment has been implicated,[7] and the same logic could be applied to anaesthetists. There is, however, an obvious conflict between the desire for a rapid turnover of cases, with a short interval between admission and surgery, and the desire for effective preoperative assessment. Patients not previously seen can be assessed in the theatre suite, imperfect though this may be, but if the solution sought is that every patient should be visited preoperatively by an anaesthetist this may be costly and pose organisational problems. If the solution sought is that every patient should be seen by his own anaesthetist this will cause considerable difficulties; the need will have to be demonstrated very clearly and changes made in hospital routine. Patients will have to be admitted to hospital earlier, operating lists definitively published at longer intervals before their scheduled time, and communication between anaesthetists and surgeons improved. This survey suggests that anaesthetists are not optimistic about the possibility of allocating more resources to achieve such changes, no matter how commendable they may be. We consider that

anaesthetists have judged the situation well, and we do not consider that any solution that costs more is justified, particularly in a climate that demands ever increasing value for money in the health service. We cannot have the best of both worlds. Limited resources mean limited services, and, although we hold differing views about preoperative assessment, we are united in the view that society as well as the profession must decide what solutions, if any, should be imposed.

c)

TABLE VI — *Value of aspects of preoperative assessment*

| | Visual analogue score* | |
Aspect	Mean	Coefficient of variation (%)
Detect potential anaesthetic problems	8·8	18
Establish rapport with patient	7·9	24
Allay patient's anxiety	7·4	31
Plan anaesthesia	7·2	35
Prescribe premedication	7·1	34
Explain anaesthesia	6·9	36
Review or order investigations	6·4	41
Detect missed pathology	6·0	46
Job satisfaction	5·7	52
Medicolegal considerations	4·6	68
Explain surgery	3·4	76

*10 = utmost important, 0 = irrelevant.

TABLE VIII — *Value of suggested methods of facilitating preopertaive assessment*

| | Visual analogue score* | |
Method	Mean	Coefficient of variation (%)
Earlier notice of surgical list	7·3	38
Earlier availability of clinical investigations	6·7	41
More cooperation from surgeons	6·4	44
Outpatient assessment clinic	5·9	49
Questionnaire completed by patient's parent	5·1	60
Questionnaire completed by patient	4·9	62
Longer admission to surgery interval	4·9	62
More anaesthetic staff	4·7	70
Decreased surgical workload	4·3	74
More cooperation from nurses	3·5	85

*10 = utmost help, 0 = no help at all.

d)

In 1978 the Association of Anaesthetists of Great Britain and Ireland received a grant from the Nuffield Provincial Hospitals Trust, which funded an inquiry into the mortality associated with anaesthesia.[1] Of the patients in that study, 8.8% did not receive a preoperative examination, suggesting that throughout the United Kingdom 300 000 patients were anaesthetised each year without previously meeting their anaesthetist. This attracted considerable publicity.[2-4] At least one book has been published discussing the preparation for anaesthesia,[5] but few reports describe actual practice. Our study investigated the practice of preoperative assessment by anaesthetists in Great Britain and Ireland.

e)

JOHN CURRAN, ANDREW T CHMIELEWSKI, JILL B WHITE, ALAN M JENNINGS

f)

References

1 Lunn JN, Mushin WW. *Mortality associated with anaesthesia*. London: Nuffield Provincial Hospitals Trust, 1982: 20.

2 Anonymous. Anaesthesia could cost 900 lives each year. *The Times* 1982 Aug 10: 2 (col 4).

3 Anonymous. Bored to death [Editorial]. *The Times* 1982 Aug 12: 12 (col 1–3).

4 Horton J. Woman's Hour. Radio 4, 1982 Sept 9. The Broadcasting Report Service, *Tellex Report:* 1–4.

5 Stevens AJ, ed. *Preparation for anaesthesia*. Tunbridge Wells: Pitman Medical, 1980.

6 Lunn JN, Mushin WW. *Mortality associated with anaesthesia*. London: Nuffield Provincial Hospitals Trust, 1982: 50.

7 Anonymous. Recipe for disaster. *Medical Defence Union Annual Report*. London: Medical Defence Union, 1984: 18.

How do the statistics given in the Abstract compare with the situation in your country?

Task 8

The reader then went on to examine the Method in greater detail. Try to complete this extract by using one word for each space.

Method

The study .... (1) started .... (2) late 1983 and completed during 1984. Members of the Anaesthetic Travelling Society and three other consultants known personally .... (3) us acted .... (4) local correspondents. Together .... (5) represented 24 departments .... (6) anaesthesia throughout Great Britain and Ireland and provided details .... (7) personnel, workload, and departmental policies that regulated preoperative assessment. .... (8) gave to each anaesthetist in their department a questionnaire .... (9) the individual's practice .... (10) preoperative assessment .... (11) in-patients undergoing elective surgery. .... (12) assessment excluded interviews .... (13) the theatre immediately .... (14) operation. .... (15) anaesthetist was asked .... (16) details .... (17) health service grade and contract, to indicate .... (18) order .... (19) frequency of use the methods by .... (20) he first gained knowledge .... (21) the clinical details of his patients, and .... (22) estimate how many of .... (23) he visited preoperatively for lists for .... (24) he was responsible. A visual analogue scale .... (25) used .... (26) evaluate suggested reasons .... (27) preoperative visiting, ... (28) factors .... (29) influenced decisions to dispense .... (30) such visits, and the improvements in organisation .... (31) might facilitate preoperative assessment.

Data .... (32) entered .... (33) a Sirius-I microcomputer .... (34) a 10 megabyte hard disc running database II software. X^2 tests .... (35) used .... (36) test for significance.

6.4   Case history: William Hudson

Role-play 2

Work in pairs. **A** should start.

A: Play the part of a surgeon. You have performed a laparotomy on Mr Hudson. You find occlusion of the superior mesenteric artery and gangrene of the small bowel. You resect most of the small bowel. Explain to Mr Hudson's son/daughter what you have done.

B: Play the part of Mr Hudson's son or daughter. Ask the surgeon about your father's operation. Ask him/her to explain the cause of your father's problem. Also ask him/her what his chances are for the future.

Unit 7   Treatment

7.1   Medical treatment

Task 1

Look back at the case of Mr Jameson (see pp. 24–5, 29, 32, 46–7, and 70) and complete as much as you can of the case notes.

SURNAME Jameson	FIRST NAMES Alan
AGE 53 SEX M	MARITAL STATUS M
OCCUPATION Carpenter	
PRESENT COMPLAINT Acute backache referred down R sciatic nerve distribution.	
O/E General Condition ENT RS CVS GIS GUS CNS	
IMMEDIATE PAST HISTORY	

What treatment would you suggest?

Task 2   🔲

Now listen to this extract from the consultation and complete the management section of the case notes.

DIAGNOSIS
MANAGEMENT

Language focus 1

Note how the doctor advises the patient about the following points:

a) the duration of the treatment:
   – *I think it will be* some weeks *before* you can go back to your kind of active work.
b) how the patient must conduct himself during the treatment:
   – *You must rest to allow* this swelling to go down . . .
   – *If you get up* . . . all the body weight above the damaged disc will press down on the disc . . .
   – *You should* also try to have your meals lying down.
   – *Don't* sit up to eat.

Practice 1   🔲

How would you advise each of these patients encountered in Unit 6?

1 A hypertensive 50-year-old director of a small company.
2 An insulin-dependent 11-year-old girl accompanied by her mother.
3 A 65-year-old schoolteacher with osteoarthritis of the left hip.
4 A 23-year-old lorry driver affected by epilepsy.
5 A 52-year-old cook with carcinoma of the bowel.
6 A 27-year-old teacher of handicapped children suffering from a depressive illness.
7 A 6-month-old baby boy suffering from atopic eczema, accompanied by his mother.

Task 3

Here is the prescription that was given to Mr Jameson.

```
┌─────────────────────────────────────────────────────────┐
│ MR  ⎫    _____                        │
│ MRS ⎪    Surname of patient-in BLOCK letters             │
│ MISS⎬                                                    │
│ Child⎭   Initials and one full forename wherever possible│
│                                                          │
│ Age if under                                             │
│ 12 years      Address                                    │
│                                             _____ │
│ YRS MTHS                                    Pharmacist's Stamp │
│ ┌──────┐  NO. OF DAYS TREATMENT         For use only by  │
│ │  NP  │  N.B. ENSURE THAT DOSE IS STATED  Pricing Bureau│
│ └──────┘                                                 │
│                                                          │
│   R                                                      │
│    x                                                     │
│        Tab. dihydrocodeine BP 30mg                       │
│        Mitte 100 (one hundred tabs)                      │
│        sig. 2 tablets, 6hrly for pain, p.c.              │
│                                                          │
│                                                          │
│                                                          │
│                                                          │
│                                                          │
│      Signature of Doctor          Date                   │
│ For use by                                               │
│ Pharmacist                                               │
│         IMPORTANT Read notes overleaf BEFORE going to the pharmacy. │
│         Medicine urgently required may be obtained outside normal │
│         hours if prescription is marked Urgent by the Doctor. │
└─────────────────────────────────────────────────────────┘
```

Which part of the prescription shows:

a) how often the tablets should be taken?
b) the purpose of the treatment?
c) the amount prescribed?
d) the name of the medicine?

What do the following abbreviations stand for?

e) Mitte
f) sig.
g) p.c.
h) tabs

Task 4 🔲

Using the information given in Task 3, try to complete the doctor's instructions to Mr Jameson.

D: Now Mr Jameson, here is a prescription for some ....(1) which you are
to take ....(2) of every ....(3) hours. Try to take them
........................(4) ....(5) if possible in case they cause you indigestion. You
........................(6) take them during the night as well if you are awake with the
........................(7).

Task 5

Try to match these treatments with the seven patients mentioned in Practice 1.

1 Tab. naproxen 250 mg
   Mitte 100
   sig. 1 tab. t.i.d.

2 Tab. imipramine 25 mg
   Mitte 100
   sig. 1 tab. t.d.s.

3 Colostomy bags
   Mitte 50

4 Human soluble insulin   Human isophane insulin
   100 IU/ml   100 IU/ml
   Mitte 10 ml × 4   Mitte 10 ml × 4
   sig. 6 IU a.m.   sig. 18 IU a.m.
        4 IU p.m.   8 IU p.m.

5 Tab. metoprolol 100 mg
   Mitte 100
   sig. 1 b.i.d.

6 Hydrocortisone cream 1%
   Mitte 30 g
   sig. apply thinly to the affected area b.i.d.

7 Tab. carbamazepine 400 mg
   Mitte 60
   sig. 1 tab. b.d.

What do the following abbreviations stand for?

a) b.i.d./b.d.
b) t.i.d./t.d.s.

Practice 2

What instructions would you give to these patients?

7.2 Physiotherapy

Task 6   [cassette]

Listen carefully to the instructions that the physiotherapist gave Mr Jameson for his spinal extension exercises. Try to put these diagrams in the correct order using the instructions. Number them 1 to 5.

a)

b)

c)

d)

e)

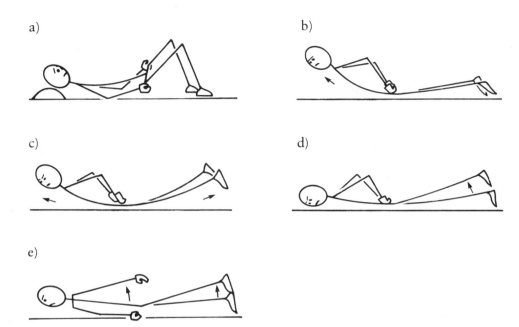

Language focus 2

Note how the physiotherapist marks the sequence of instructions:
– *First of all* you lie down . . .
– *Now* place your hands on your back . . .

Read through the Tapescript for Task 6 and underline the markers of sequence used.

Note how the physiotherapist advises the patient:
– You *should* do these exercises three times a day, *preferably* on an empty stomach.
– You *should try to do* them as slowly and smoothly as possible . . .

For precautions she says:
– You should *try to avoid* jerking your body.

Practice 3

Complete the advice and precautions given to Mr Jameson using appropriate language.

1 .... on a hard surface.

2 .... careful while getting out of bed.

.... roll over and then get up from your side.

3 .... bending forward, for example if you are picking up something off the floor.

4 .... to bend your knees and keep your back straight.

5 .... lifting heavy weights.

Practice 4

Using the diagrams in Task 6 as cues, instruct and advise Mr Jameson on his spinal extension exercises. Remember to use sequence markers and the correct verb forms.

7.3   Surgical treatment

Practice 5

Mr Jameson's condition has worsened and his doctor has decided to refer him to a neurosurgeon. Using the cues below and the language that you have studied in this and earlier units, explain the decision to Mr Jameson.

1 Sympathise with the patient about the continuing pain and the development of weakness in the patient's right foot.
2 Explain that this weakness is due to continued pressure on the nerve roots supplying the muscles of his leg.
3 Explain that the pressure is at the level of the disc between the lumbar vertebrae.
4 Explain that you think he should be referred to a neurosurgeon and why.
5 Reassure the patient about the operation and follow-up treatment.
6 Explain the prognosis if the patient agrees to the operation.
7 Explain the prognosis if the patient doesn't have the operation.
8 Ask the patient if there are any further points he would like explained.

Task 7

Study the Medications section of this Discharge Summary. Transfer this summary of the patient's medication to the Hospital Prescription Sheet.

THE ROYAL INFIRMARY   **DISCHARGE SUMMARY:**

To: Dr Winton
Cardiologist
Southern General

Dr Wallace
High Street
Everton

Date of admission: 30.8.85 & 15.9.85 (SGH)
Date of discharge: 5.9.85 & 24.9.85 (Memorial)
Ward: 14
Consultant: Mr A. Swan

| Surname: Wynne | Forenames: John | Number: 1563526 |

Address: 5 Nelson Street, Everton

Principal diagnosis: Crescendo angina
? recent myocardial infarct

Principal operation: CAVG X 4,
single saph grafts to LAD,
RCA, sequential saph graft to
OM1 and OM2

Other conditions:

Date of operation: 17.9.85

Other operations

External cause of injury

PM/no PM	Tumour type	Histological verification of tumour type	Verified/Not verified

HISTORY: 58-year-old car salesman who has been hypertensive for 15 years. Had an inferior myocardial infarction in 1981. For the past 3 months he has had increasing angina pectoris which has been present at rest. Recently admitted to hospital with prolonged chest pain, found to have positive thallium scan despite negative acute ECG or enzyme changes. Other past history of hypothyriodism diagnosed 3 years ago. Stopped smoking 20 cigarettes a day 5 years ago.

MEDICATIONS: Aspirin 300 mg daily, GTN transdermal patch 1 daily, Minihep 5000 units t.d.s., diamorphine 5 mg 4 hourly p.r.n., cyclizine 50 mg 4 hourly p.r.n., paracetamol 1 g q.d.s., temazepam 20 mg nocte, GTN p.r.n., atenolol 100 mg daily, isosorbide mononitrate 40 mg b.d., thyroxine 0.1 mg daily, bendrofluazide/potassium chloride tablet daily nifedipine 20 mg t.d.s.

EXAMINATION: Obese. Pulse 60 regular, BP 130/80, no signs of failure, heart sounds normal. Soft midsystolic murmur at apex and aortic areas.

INVESTIGATIONS: Routine haematology and biochemistry normal. Chest X-ray: normal. ECG showed evidence of previous infarct, Q waves in T_3 + AVF, inverted T_5 in V_1 - V_5.

PRESCRIPTION SHEET

Sheet No. .... *Please use a ball point pen*

ORAL and OTHER NON-PARENTERAL MEDICINES – REGULAR PRESCRIPTIONS

CODE	Date Com-menced	MEDICINES (Block Letters)	DOSE	Method of Admin.	AM 6	AM 8	AM 10	MD 12	PM 2	PM 6	PM 10	MN 12	Other Times	DOCTOR'S SIGNATURE	Discontinued Date	Discontinued Initials
								Times of Administration								
A																
B																
C																
D																
E																
F																
G																
H																
I																
J																
K																
L																

PARENTERAL MEDICINES – REGULAR PRESCRIPTIONS

CODE																
M																
N																
O																
P																
Q																

ORAL and OTHER NON-PARENTERAL MEDICINES – ONCE ONLY PRESCRIPTIONS

Date	MEDICINE	DOSE	Method of Admin.	Time of Admin.*	DOCTOR'S SIGNATURE	Given by Initials	Time if Diff.*

PARENTERAL MEDICINES – ONCE ONLY PRESCRIPTIONS

Date	MEDICINE	DOSE	Method of Admin.	Time of Admin.*	DOCTOR'S SIGNATURE	Given by Initials	Time if Diff.*

NAME OF PATIENT	AGE	UNIT NUMBER	CONSULTANT

KNOWN DRUG/MEDICINE SENSITIVITY

PLEASE ✓ WHEN MEDICINES ARE PRESCRIBED ON

Fluid (Additive Medicine) Prescription Chart	
Diabetic Chart	
Anticoagulant Chart	
Anaesthetic Prescription Sheet	
Record of Labour Sheet	

If medicine discontinued because of suspected adverse reaction please enter in box below

	MEDICINE	ADVERSE REACTION
1		
2		

DIET

Date	DETAILS	Initials

Task 8

Study this extract from the Procedure Section. It is taken from page 2 of the Discharge Summary. Complete the gaps in the procedure using these verbs. The verbs are not in the correct order.

administered   cross-clamped
prepared   continued
anastomosed   rewarmed
grafted   opened

PROCEDURE: Vein was .... (1) for use as grafts. Systemic
             heparin was .... (2) and bypass established,
the left ventricle was vented, the aorta was .... (3)
and cold cardioplegic arrest of the heart obtained. Topical cooling
was .... (4) for the duration of the aortic cross clamp.
   Attention was first turned to the first and second obtuse marginal
branches of the circumflex coronary artery. The first obtuse marginal
was intramuscular with proximal artheroma. It admitted a 1.5 mm
occluder and was .... (5) with saphenous sequential grafts,
side to side using continuous 6/0 special prolene which was used
for all subsequent distal anastomoses. The end of this saphenous
graft was recurved and .... (6) to the second obtuse
marginal around a 1.75 mm occluder.
   The left anterior descending was .... (7) in its distal
half and accepted a 1.5 mm occluder around which it was grafted
with a single length of long saphenous vein.
   Lastly, the right coronary artery was opened at the crux and
again grafted with a single length of saphenous vein around a
1.5 mm occluder whilst the circulation was .... (8).

CLOSURE:

Complete Task 9 before you check your answers in the Key.

Task 9

Put these steps in the correct sequence to show how the operation was completed. Step 1 is (a) and step 7 is (g). The other steps are out of sequence.

a) Release aortic cross-clamp and vent air from the left heart and ascending aorta.
b) Administer protamine sulphate and adjust blood volume.
c) Defibrillate the heart and wean heart off bypass.
d) Remove cannulae and repair cannulation and vent sites.
e) Complete proximal vein anastomoses to the ascending aorta.
f) Ascertain haemostasis.
g) Insert drains.

When you have ordered them correctly, write your own version of the final section of the procedure notes like this:

– *The aortic cross-clamp was released and air vented from the left heart and ascending aorta.*

Check your answers to this task and Task 8 using page 2 of the Discharge Summary in the Key.

Task 10

Using page 2 of the Discharge Summary in the Key, work out the meaning of these abbreviations.

1 CAVG
2 LAD
3 RCA
4 OM1
5 LV

Task 11

Explain in simple terms to the patient the purpose of this operation and how you will accomplish it.

7.4   Reading skills: using an index

Task 12

Here is the inside cover page from *Current Contents*. Scan the page to find out:

— what it is;
— where it is published;
— how often it is published;
— the address through which you would be able to order it.

CURRENT CONTENTS®

Life Sciences

(ISSN 0011-3409)

A PRODUCT OF THE
INSTITUTE FOR SCIENTIFIC INFORMATION®, INC.
EUGENE GARFIELD
PRESIDENT
PETER K. ABORN
SENIOR VICE PRESIDENT & GENERAL MANAGER
CURRENT AWARENESS PRODUCTS DIVISION
BEVERLY BARTOLOMEO
DIRECTOR, CURRENT CONTENTS
MARYANN CHAPPELL
MANAGER, CURRENT CONTENTS

WHAT IS *CURRENT CONTENTS*?

Current Contents is your own personal library of over 1,130 of the world's most important journals. It gives you access to the tables of contents of the latest journal issues published and saves you valuable time locating information vital to your professional needs.

The compact weekly editions can be carried with you anywhere and read whenever you have a minute to spare. The easy to scan format helps you keep on top of more than 228,000 journal and book articles published each year in the life sciences.

Each *CC®* issue contains these weekly features:

Current Book Contents® highlights the tables of contents of new, multi-authored books. It provides complete bibliographic information and includes an easy to use order coupon.

Title Word Index lists all significant words, translated into English, from every article title appearing that week. It enables you to quickly locate articles on a given topic.

Author Index & Address Directory supplies the names and addresses of authors to contact for reprint requests.

Publishers Address Directory lists the names and addresses of the publishers whose journals are covered that week in *CC*, providing the information you need to contact the journal for subscription information.

CC regularly publishes these additional features:

Triannual Cumulative Journal Index enables you to locate every journal issue published in *CC* during a four month period. The index refers you to the *CC* issue and page number on which the table of contents of each journal issue appeared.

List of Serials & Publishers Guide provides you with a complete list of the journals and books covered. It is published twice a year; copies are available from *ISI®* upon request.

HOW TO OBTAIN ARTICLES LISTED IN CC:

ISI offers a fast, efficient document delivery service, *OATS® (Original Article Text Service)*. OATS orders can be placed by mail; telephone (215-386-4399); telex (84-5305); facsimile machine; or online through DIALOG, SDC, CLASS, or the *ISI* Search Network. If you wish to write for reprints, you can locate the author's address in the **Author Index & Address Directory**.

CUSTOMER SERVICE

For subscription information and address changes, contact Laura Weissenberg, Manager, Customer Services.

For editorial questions concerning *CC*, contact Beverly Bartolomeo, Director, *Current Contents*.

Write *ISI*, 3501 Market Street, Philadelphia, PA. 19104 or phone toll-free 800-523-1850 in US (except PA.) or (215) 386-0100/Cable: SCINFO/Telex: 84-5305.

HOW TO ORDER

United States: One year (52 weekly issues) $245. **Canada & Mexico:** $285. **Central & South America:** $375. **Europe & Mideast (except F.R.G. & Austria)** $285. **F.R.G. & Austria:** 757 DM. **All Others:** Rates available on request. Air mail delivery of *CC* is also available. For complete mailing and ordering information (including information about special group rates) contact the *ISI* office, agent or representative nearest you:

In the **U.S.** contact: Director of Subscriptions, *ISI*, 3501 Market Street, Philadelphia, PA. 19104. Telephone toll-free 800-523-1850 in U.S. (except PA.) or (215) 386-0100/Cable: SCINFO/Telex: 84-5305.

In **Canada** contact: *ISI*, 566 Church Street, Toronto, Ontario M4Y 2E3. Phone: (416) 922-0608.

In **Federal Republic of Germany & Austria** contact: *ISI*, GmbH, Stadthof 9, 6050 OFFENBACH AM MAIN, Federal Republic of Germany. Phone: 0611-889077.

Elsewhere in Europe, N. Africa & Middle East contact: *ISI*, 132 High Street, UXBRIDGE, Middlesex UB8 1DP, U.K. Phone: 44-895-30085. Telex: 933693 UKISI.

In **India & Bangladesh** contact: Universal Subscription Agency Pvt. Ltd., 117/H-1/294-B, Model Town, Pandu Nagar. Kanpur-208025. India. Phone: 81300. Cable: WORLDMAGS (Kanpur). Telex: 31-3916 (Delhi).

In **Japan** contact: USACO Corporation (formerly U.S. Asiatic Co., Ltd.), Tsutsumi Building, 13-12 Shimbashi, 1-chome, Minato-ku, Tokyo 105, Japan. Phone: (03) 502-6471, Telex: USACO J26274, or Kinokuniya Co., Ltd., 17-7 Shinjuku, 3-chome, Shinjuku-ku, Tokyo 160-91, Japan. Phone: (03) 354-0131, Telex: 0234759 KINOKU J.

In **Taiwan** contact: Good Faith Worldwide International Co. Ltd., 9th Floor #118, Section 2, Chung Hsiao E. Road, Taipei, Taiwan 100. Phone: (02) 3917396, 3917397, 3964720. Telex: 11862 GDFH.

In **Latin America** contact: Ing. J. Robles G., Apartado 19-202, Mexico D.F., Mexico 03910. Phone: 680-5271.

In **Asia, Australia & New Zealand** contact: R.T. Tanner, 7 Mei Hwan View #03-08, Singapore 2056, Republic of Singapore. Phone: 283-4181.

Current Contents is mailed every week on the same day except holidays when it is mailed one or more days earlier. If delivery is irregular in any way, please check local postal services.

The *Institute for Scientific Information* makes a reasonable effort to supply complete and accurate information in its information services, but does not assume any liability for errors or omissions.

ISI will fill claims for missing issues of *Current Contents* if received within three months of cover date.

Second-Class Postage Paid at Philadelphia, PA.

Statement of frequency: Weekly

POSTMASTER: Send address changes to Subscription Manager, *Current Contents*, Institute for Scientific Information, Inc., 3501 Market Street, Philadelphia, PA 19104, USA.

©Copyright 1984 by the

ISI®

Institute for Scientific Information®, Inc.
3501 Market Street
Philadelphia, Pennsylvania 19104, USA

Task 13

Here is the Index of Journals that featured in *Current Contents* (18 June 1984).

If you were interested in articles concerned with renal transplants/transplantation, which journals might you think of consulting? Note down the titles and the *Current Contents* page references.

Task 14

Here is the relevant page from the Subject Index at the back of *Current Contents*.

What do you think the following abbreviations stand for?

CC Pg   J Pg

Task 15

Use the Subject Index to check whether any of the journals that you listed for Task 13 are referred to. (Check the CC Pg references against your list.) Also note down the J Pg references.

Task 16

You decide to consult the Contents Page for *Transplantation*. On which page of *Current Contents* would you find it?

(SR774)   **Transplantation**   Williams & Wilkins Co.
Abstracts in English

VOL. 37 NO. 5   MAY 1984

CURRENT CONTENTS® © 1984 by ISI®   LS, V. 27 #25, June 18, 1984   133

Task 17

List the titles referred to in the Subject Index.

Task 18

Here are the abstracts from a selection of articles on the same subject. Can you match any of them to the titles given in the Contents Page of *Transplantation*?

1   **Kidney and patient survival of 351 consecutive patients undergoing first cadaveric renal transplants since 1968 were reviewed to determine the effects of splenectomy on outcome. Special emphasis was given to analysis of 106 splenectomized and 102 nonsplenectomized patients treated since 1975. During the first two years after transplant, kidney survival was better in the splenectomized patients, with no adverse effect on patient survival. However, after the first two years, patient survival became significantly worse in splenectomized patients (35.5% vs. 60.5% at 84 months). Of the deaths, infection was the cause in 26.7% of nonsplenectomized patients compared with 50% of splenectomized patients ($P<0.07$). Of patients alive at one year posttransplant, death rates were not different in patients splenectomized before 1975 or after 1975. Timing of splenectomy (prior vs. concurrent) had no effect on outcome. The adverse effect of splenectomy on mortality appeared to be more pronounced in younger (≤45 year-old) than in older (>45 year-old) patients. Splenectomy should not be performed routinely in preparation for a cadaveric transplant because of an unacceptably high late mortality that is primarily from sepsis.**

2

A retrospective study of 410 renal transplant recipients showed that 1.96% (8/410) of patients had developed severe non-typhoid salmonella infections. The clinical features seen were fever, leucopenia, pneumonia, diarrhoea, abscesses, pyelonephritis, venous thrombosis and pleural effusion. Neither uraemia nor repeated high doses of steroids seemed to be major precipitating events. All isolates were strains of *Salmonella entiritidis*. All 8 patients were cured and none became permanent carriers. Salmonella infections cause severe, life-threatening infections in renal transplant patients and require vigorous treatment often with a long-term low-dose regimen. Patients seemed to respond best to chloramphenicol, but ampicillin and co-trimoxazole were useful in some. Bilateral nephrectomy should be performed before the transplantation if the organism is grown from the urine.

3   Sera of 154 recipients of renal allografts were studied for transplantation heterophile (T-H) antibodies by means of immunodiffusion, mixed agglutination (MA) and enzyme immunoassay (EIA). T-H antibodies were found by immunodiffusion against bovine red blood cell (BRBC) extracts (15%) and sheep red blood cell (SRBC) extracts (12%): The specificity of antibodies to BRBC was shown to be distinct from that of antibodies to SRBC. Both of these T-H antibody types were absorbable by guinea pig kidney (GPK) tissue sediments and, therefore, they could be classified into the GPK-positive group of heterophile antibodies. The MA test was successfully employed to demonstrate directly T-H antibodies combining with antigens of GPK. Results of the MA inhibition studies and those of EIA indicated that some of the BRBC antibodies are directed to antigens of asialo-high molecular-weight glycoprotein of BRBC.

4   The relation between urinary kallikrein excretion (Ukal) and rejection, graft function, and blood pressure was studied in 45 renal transplant recipients. Ukal was assayed by means of an enzymatic (amidolytic) method, as well as with a specific radioimmunoassay. In a group of 10 patients studied longitudinally from the day of transplantation till day 35±3, an increase in urinary amidolytic activity without a concomitant increase in kallikrein antigen excretion was found to precede 11 out of 14 rejection episodes. This increased amidolytic activity generally persisted for several days. It was demonstrated by chromatography using an immunoadsorbent column of antiurokallikrein that the rejection-associated esterase, or esterases, differed from urokallikrein.

In 35 outpatient recipients with stable graft function, Ukal excretion was decreased compared with that of healthy controls (42±7.5 vs. 107.5±7.3 μg/24 hr by radioimmunoassay and 0.70±0.08 vs. 1.10±0.07 U/24 hr, using the amidolytic method); for these patients a significant correlation between Ukal excretion and creatinine clearance was found ($P<0.02$). Both in transplant recipients and in controls there was a close correlation between the results of the two Ukal assays ($P<0.001$). No significant relation between Ukal excretion and blood pressure was found, either for patients or for controls. It is concluded that acute graft rejection is accompanied by an increased excretion of nonurokallikrein esterase(s). The lower Ukal excretion in patients with stable renal function seems to be related to their reduced renal function. No relation between Ukal excretion and blood pressure levels was found.

Tapescript

Unit 1 Taking a history I

Task 1

D: Good morning, Mr Hall. What's brought you along today?
P: Well you see doctor, I've been having these headaches, you see, and . . .
D: And how long have they been bothering you?
P: Well they started about, well it must have been about three months ago.
D: I see. And which part of your head is affected?
P: Well, it's, it's right across the front here.
D: And, can you describe the pain?
P: It's a sort of dull, dull and throbbing kind of pain.
D: I see, and, do they come on at any particular time?
P: They seem to be, they're usually worse in the morning. I notice them when I wake up.
D: And is there anything that makes them better?
P: Well, if I lie down for a while, they seem to get, they go away.
D: Yes, and has there been anything else apart from these headaches?
P: Well, the wife, my wife, she says that I seem to be getting a bit deaf.
D: Well Mr Hall, I think at this stage I'll start by checking your ears to see if there's any wax . . .

Task 4

D: Come in, Mr Green. Come and sit down here. I've had a letter from your doctor and he tells me that you've been having pain, pain in your chest.
P: Yes, and in my arm, and also tingling in my fingers and . . .
D: Yes, now when did you first notice this pain?
P: Well, I suppose about six months ago.
D: And can you remember when it first came on?
P: Yes, well I remember, I got a bad pain in my chest when I was shopping. It was so bad I couldn't breathe and . . .
D: And where, in which part of your chest did you feel the pain?
P: Right across my chest.
D: And how long did it last?
P: About ten minutes.
D: And what did you do when it happened?
P: I had to stop and, wait for it to go away.
D: So, have you had this, the pain again since then?
P: Yes, I often get it when I overdo things, and when I . . .
D: Well, I think at this stage I'd like to examine you, your chest. So if you could strip to your waist. Fine. I'll just check your pulse first of all. Fine. That's fine. It's quite normal, seventy per minute. Now your blood pressure. Fine. That's quite normal too. 130 over 80.
P: I'm pleased to hear it.

D: Now I'm going to listen to your heart, so I want you to breathe normally. Your heart sounds quite normal.

P: Well, that's a relief.

D: Well now, I want you to take deep breaths in and out while I check your lungs. In. Out. In. Out. Fine. They're completely clear. Well Mr Green, the pain you've been having sounds very like the pain of what we call angina, and this, this occurs when not enough oxygen is getting to the heart. I'd like to check a few tests, and, following that I'll be able to advise some treatment for you . . .

Task 6

D: Ah good morning Mr Hudson. I see from your card that you've just moved into the area and perhaps you could tell me a little about your previous health as I won't get your records for another month, month or two, and then we can deal with your present problem.

P: Well I've actually, I've always been very fit up till now but . . .

D: Have you ever been in hospital?

P: Only when I was a child. I had an appendicitis when I was eight.

D: And what's your job, what do you do?

P: Well, I'm a, I work for the post office. I'm a postmaster.

D: And I see that you're what, 58, now, and have you . . .?

P: Yes.

D: Have you always been with the post office?

P: Yes, well apart from my time in the army you know . . .

D: I see. And you're married. Any family?

P: Yes, two girls and a boy.

D: Fine. That's fine. Now can you tell me what seems to be the problem today?

P: Well, it's this terrible pain. I've got this terrible pain in my back. I've had it for more than a week now and it's . . .

D: I see, and can you show me exactly where it is?

P: It's down here, here.

D: And does it go anywhere else?

P: Yes, it goes down my left leg. And I feel pins and needles in my foot.

D: I see, and is it there all the time?

P: Yes, yes it is. It's keeping me awake, awake at night and I can't get out into the garden. I've been taking aspirins but the pain, it just comes back again.

D: And was there anything that started it off?

P: Well yes, yes. I've been trying to sort out the garden at my new house and I don't know, I may have been overdoing things a bit.

Unit 2 Taking a history II

Tasks 1 and 2

D: Now Mrs Brown, can you tell me, have you any trouble with your stomach or bowels?
P: Well, I sometimes get a bit of indigestion.
D: I see, and could you tell me more about that?
P: Well, it only comes on if I have a hot, something spicy, you know, like a curry.
D: I see, well that's quite normal really. And what's your appetite like?
P: Not bad.
D: And any problems with your waterworks?
P: No, they're, they're all right.
D: And are you still having your periods regularly?
P: No, they stopped, must have been five years ago.
D: Any pain in the chest, any palpitations, swelling of the ankles?
P: Not really doctor.
D: And what about coughs or wheezing or shortness of breath?
P: Only when I've got a cold.
D: Have you noticed any weakness or tingling in your limbs?
P: No, no I can't say that I have really.
D: What sort of mood have you been in recently?
P: I've been feeling a bit down. You know, I'm not sleeping well.

Task 3 and Language focus 2

D: And how long, how long have you had this temperature?
P: Oh, I don't know exactly. About two months on and off.
D: And does, is the temperature there all the time or does it come on at any particular time?
P: Well, sometimes I'm all right during the day but, I wake up at night and I'm drenched in sweat, drenched, and sometimes my whole body shakes and . . .
D: And how have you been feeling in general?
P: Well, I don't know, I've been feeling a bit tired, a bit tired and weak. And I just don't seem to have any energy.
D: And have you noticed any, any pain in your muscles?
P: Yes, well actually I have a bit, yes.
D: And what about your weight. Have you lost any weight?
P: Yes, yes I have, about a stone.*
D: I see, and, what about your appetite. What's your appetite been like?
P: Well, I've really been off my food this last while. I just haven't felt like eating.
D: And have you had a cough at all?
P: Oh yes, I have. Nearly all the time. I sometimes bring up a lot of phlegm.
D: And is there, have you noticed any blood in it?
P: No, not always but yes, sometimes.
D: Have you had any pains in your chest?
P: Only if I take a deep breath.

---

* In the UK patients often talk about their weight in stones.
   1 stone = 14 pounds or 6.4 kg.
   1 pound = 454 grams.
   In the USA, people give their weight in pounds.

Tasks 11 and 12

D: Good afternoon, Mr Hudson. Just have a seat. I haven't seen you for a good long time. What's brought you along here today?

P: Well doctor. I've been having these headaches and I seem to have lost some weight, and ...

D: I see, and how long have these headaches been bothering you?

P: Well, I don't know. For quite a while now. The wife passed away you know, about four months ago. And I've been feeling down since then.

D: And which part of your head is affected?

P: Just here. Just here on the top. It feels as if there were something heavy, a heavy weight pressing down on me.

D: I see, and have they affected your vision at all?

P: No, no I wouldn't say so.

D: Not even seeing lights or black spots?

P: No, nothing like that.

D: And they haven't made you feel sick at all?

P: No.

D: Now you told me that you've lost some weight. What's your appetite been like?

P: Well actually I haven't really been feeling like eating. I've really been off my food for the moment and ...

D: And what about your bowels, any problems?

P: No, no they're, I'm quite all right, no problems.

D: And what about your waterworks?

P: Well, I've been having trouble getting started and I have to, I seem to have to get up during the night, two or three times at night.

D: And has this come on recently?

P: Well, no, not exactly. I think I've noticed it gradually over the past, the past few months.

D: And do you get any pain when you're passing water?

P: No, no.

D: And have you noticed any blood, any traces of blood?

P: No, no, I can't say that I have.

Unit 3   Examining a patient

Task 1

D: Would you slip off your top things, please. Now I just want to see you standing. Hands by your side. You're sticking that hip out a little bit, aren't you?

P: Yes, well, I can't straighten up easily.

D: Could you bend down as far as you can with your knees straight and stop when you have had enough?

P: Oh, that's the limit.

D: Not very far, is it? Stand up again. Now I would like you to lean backwards. That's not much either. Now stand straight up again. Now first of all I would like you to slide your right hand down the right side of your thigh. See how far you can go. That's fine. Now do the same thing on the opposite side. Fine. Now just come back to standing straight. Now keep your feet together just as they are. Keep your knees firm. Now try and turn both shoulders round to the right. Look right round. Keep your knees and feet steady.

P: Oh, that's sore.

D: Go back to the centre again. Now try the same thing and go round to the left side. Fine. Now back to the centre. That's fine. Now would you like to get on to the couch and lie on your face? I'm just going to find out where the sore spot is.

Task 2 and Practice 1

D: Would you like to lie down here on the couch, on your back?

P: OK.

D: I'm going to test your reflexes by tapping you with this little hammer. It won't hurt you. Let me hold your right arm. Let it go quite relaxed. Try not to tighten up. There. Now the other one. Just let me have your wrist. Let it go quite floppy. That's right. I'm going to tap your elbow. Fine. Now the left one. OK?

P: Fine.

D: I'll just give you a little tap here on the wrist. Now the other one. Now let your legs go completely relaxed. I'll hold them up with my hand. There. I'm just going to turn your leg out to the side for a moment. Just relax. That's it. Now the other one. Fine.

Task 4

D: Now Mr McLeod, I know you're in some pain but there are a few things I'll have to check. I'll be as quick as I can. I'll just take your pulse. Now the other side. OK. Now your blood pressure. You've had that done before. I'm going to check the other side too. Once more. Fine. Now I want to listen to your heart. Just breathe normally. Could you sit up a little? I just want to check your lungs.

P: Right doctor.

D: That's it. Now I'd like you to take big breaths in and out through your mouth. OK. You can lie down again.

P: It's bad.

D: I'll be quick. I'll just take a look at your stomach. Take deep breaths in and out. Now I'm going to check the pulses in your groins too. We'll just roll your pyjama trousers down. That's it. We're finished now. Well Mr McLeod, I think you've got some trouble with one of your arteries because of your high blood pressure. I'll give you an injection to relieve the pain and arrange for you to go into hospital for further tests.

Unit 4   Special examinations

Tasks 1, 2 and 3

D: Good afternoon Mr Priestly, come in and have a seat.

P: Good afternoon Mr Davidson.

D: Now I've had a letter from your doctor saying that you've been having problems with your sight.

P: Yes, that's right doctor.

D: Could you tell me how long the left eye has been bad for?

P: Oh, going on for about a year now I suppose.

D: And what do you do?

P: I'm a postman. I deliver letters and that sort of thing.

D: How is your work being affected?

P: Oh it's really bad. I can hardly see the letters let alone the addresses. I have to get my mates to do that sort of thing for me and it's getting to a stage where I just can't cope really.

D: I see, yes. I'd just like to examine your eyes and perhaps we could start with the chart. Could you just look at the chart for me? Can you see any letters at all?

P: No, nothing.

D: OK. Well with the right eye can you see anything?

P: N H T A, that's about all I'm afraid.

D: Now does that make any difference?

P: No, no nothing.

D: What about that one, does that have any effect?

P: Not really, I can't really say it does.

D: Right, OK, thank you very much indeed.

Tasks 4 and 5

D: Now Debbie, can I have a look at you to find out where your bad cough is coming from?

P: (*Nods*)

D: Would you like to stay sitting on Mum's knee?

P: (*Nods*)

D: That's fine. Now let's ask Mum to take off your jumper and blouse. You'll not be cold in here. (*Mother removes Debbie's clothes*) Now I'm going to put this thing on your chest. It's called a stethoscope. It might be a bit cold. I'll warm it up. Feel the end there. OK? First of all I listen to your front and then your back.

Mother: She's had that done lots of times by Dr Stuart.

D: Good, well done. You didn't move at all. Now I'd like to see your tummy, so will you lie on the bed for a minute? Will I guess what's in your tummy this morning? I bet it's Rice Krispies.

P: (*Nods*)

⟫→

D: Now while you're lying there, I'll feel your neck and under your arms. Are you tickly? Now the top of your legs. That's all very quick, isn't it? Mrs Thomson, could Debbie sit on your knee again? I'd like you to hold her there while I examine her ears and throat. Right, Debbie. Here's a little light to look in your ears. This will tickle a bit but won't be sore. Good girl. What a nice ear. Now let's see the other one. Now nearly the last bit. Open your mouth. Let me see your teeth. Now open it as wide as you can. Good. I wonder how tall you are Debbie. Could you come and stand over here and I'll measure you? Stand straight. That's fine. Have you ever been on a weighing machine? Just stand up here and we'll see how heavy you are. Well, we're all finished now. You've been very good. I'll have a talk with your Mum and you can play with the toys for a minute.

Tasks 7, 8 and 9

D: Hello Mr Walters. How are you today?

P: Oh I'm fine, very well thank you.

D: You know who I am don't you?

P: Now let me see now. I know your face, but I don't quite place who you are. I think I know. I think I should know who you are.

D: Well that's right. I'm Dr Watson. I've met you several times before you know.

P: Oh you're the doctor. Well I remember old Dr Horsburgh quite well. I remember when he had a surgery down in the old Kirkgate. but I don't remember seeing him recently.

D: No, Dr Horsburgh's been retired for a good number of years now. I took over his practice and I've seen you before. Maybe you don't recall that. Have you been here long?

P: Where, where do you mean?

D: In this house, have you been here long?

P: Oh I've been here some time I think.

D: Do you remember where this is? Where is this place?

P: This'll be the High Street isn't it?

D: Yes this is the High Street. How long have you been living in the High Street?

P: Oh it must be a good number of years now. I, my mother used to stay down in North High Street of course, and I used to stay with her, but when I got married I moved up here. Oh that must be a good number of years. I can't quite remember the time.

D: Do you remember when you were born? What was the year of your birth? Can you remember that?

P: Oh yes. I was born in 1902.

D: Oh what month were you born in? Do you remember that?

P: Oh yes. I'm an April baby. I was always an April baby. Not an April fool, not the 1st of April you know.

D: Do you remember what time of the month? What was the date?

P: Oh it was the 17th of April.

D: Well how old will you be now, do you think?

P: Oh I've retired now. I must be about 69 I think. I'll be about 69.

D: Well there's no doubt the years go by. What year is it this year? Do you know that?

P: Well this'll be about 1978 now I suppose.

D: Fine, and what month are we in?

P: Oh now let me see. It'll be, the, I can't, can't remember doctor.

D: Well tell me, is it summer or winter?

P: Oh well I suppose it's so cold it must be the winter time. It'll be January. Is that right?

D: Well actually it's February now, but it feels as though it was January, doesn't it? Do you remember what day of the week it is? Or do the days not mean a great deal to you now that you're not working?

P: Oh you're right the days seem to run into each other, but this'll be Tuesday, I think. No, no it'll be Wednesday isn't it?

D: Well I suppose that Wednesday or Thursday, one day tends to become much the same as the other when we're not working. Isn't that right?

P: Oh you're right there.

D: Well I wonder if you could do this other little test for me. This is really some common things I'd like you to think about and tell me the answer for. It's to do with this last illness you had and it's to help me decide how you're progressing and if we need to give you any different kind of medical treatment.

P: All right. I don't mind. Anything to help you.

Task 10, Language focus 4 and Task 11

Part 1

D: I now want to test how well you can feel things on the skin. I'm going to ask you to close your eyes and say 'yes' each time you feel me touching the skin of your legs with this small piece of cotton wool. I'll touch the back of your hand with it now. Do you feel that?

P: Yes doctor.

D: Well every time you feel me touch your legs say 'yes'.

Part 2

D: Well that was quite easy wasn't it? Now I'm going to try something a little different. I have this sharp needle with this blunt end. I want you to say 'sharp' or 'blunt' each time you feel me touch.

Part 3

D: The other sensation I want to test is whether you feel this tube hot or this other tube which is cold. Remember I want you to keep your eyes closed, and each time I touch the skin of your legs I want you to tell me whether it is hot or cold.

Part 4

D: Next I'm going to test you with this vibrating fork. I'm going to press it on the ankle bone and I want you to tell me whether you feel it vibrating, and if you do, to say 'stop' when you feel it has stopped.

Part 5

D: I'm now going to test the pulses in your legs. First we'll press on the blood vessel here in the groin. And now behind the knee. Could you bend it a little for me? And here behind the ankle bone. And now the top of the foot. And now the other leg.

Unit 5   Investigations

Task 2

D: Now I'm going to take some fluid off your back to find out what is giving you these headaches. Nurse will help me. It won't take very long. Now I want you to move right to the edge of the bed. That's it. Right. Lie on your left side. Now can you bend both your knees up as far as they will go? I'll just put a pillow between your knees to keep you comfortable. Put your head down to meet your knees, curl up. I'm going to wipe your back with some antiseptic. You'll feel it a bit cold. Now I'm going to give you a local anaesthetic so it won't be sore. You'll feel just a slight jab, OK? We'll wait for a few minutes for that to take effect. Right now, lie still, that's very important.

Task 3 (Three doctors – A, B and C)

A: An ECG is essential because it will show any changes in the heart: axis, ischaemia, left ventricular hypertrophy.

B: I think a chest X-ray is also very important to see the size of the heart and the extent of any hypertrophy. I would also check the creatinine to see if there's any damage to the kidneys.

C: An intravenous pyelogram is essential because a renal cause is very likely.

B: As an initial investigation?

C: No, after urea and electrolytes and after the creatinine.

B: It's essential *if* the creatinine shows something wrong with the kidneys.

C: Yes.

A: Yes, both creatinine and urea and electrolytes are required. In this case I think they're more important than the ECG and chest X-ray because the patient is young, 43, and the hypertension is very high.

C: Urine analysis too in this case. It's very important.

B: Yes, it's routine.

C: We can see if there's any glomerular damage. We may find blood, albumin, casts ...

A: Yes, it's very important.

B: What about radioisotope studies of the kidneys?

C: Not essential, but we could do this to check the function of the kidneys.

A: We can see this from the creatinine and urine.

C: I know. It's not essential, but it could be useful.

B: Serum cholesterol?

A: Not essential. We're thinking of another type of hypertension here. But possibly useful.

B: Skull X-ray?

C: Not required. It's of no value in this case.

B: Serum thyroxine?

A: Absolutely no connection with hypertension.

B: Barium meal?

C: Not required.

B: Uric acid?

A: Not necessary. If the uric acid is raised, there would be other symptoms.

Task 4

Lab Tech:	This is the haematology lab at the Royal. I have a result for you.
D:	Right. I'll just get a form. OK.
Lab Tech:	It's for Mr Hall, Mr Kevin Hall.
D:	Right.
Lab Tech:	White blood cells, seven point two; RBC, three point three two; haemoglobin, twelve point nine. That's twelve point nine. Haematocrit, point three nine; MCV, eighty-one; platelets, two six four.
D:	Sorry?
Lab Tech:	Two six four, two hundred and sixty-four.
D:	Right.
Lab Tech:	ESR, forty-three millimetres.
D:	OK. I've got that.
Lab Tech:	Blood film showed, neutrophils, sixty per cent; lymphocytes, thirty per cent; monocytes, five per cent; eosinophils, four per cent; basophils, one per cent.
D:	Fine. Anything else on the film?
Lab Tech:	Yes, there are burr cells present plus plus.
D:	Right. Thanks very much.

Unit 6   Making a diagnosis

Tasks 1 and 2

D: Hello Mr Nicol, I haven't seen you for a long time. What seems to be the problem?
P: I have been having these headaches, doctor.
D: Which part of your head?
P: Mostly along here, along this side.
D: Oh I see, the left side. How long have they been bothering you?
P: Well they started about three weeks ago. At first I felt as if I had the flu because my shoulders were aching, you know pains in the joints and I had a bit of a temperature.
D: I see, and did you take anything for the headaches?
P: I took some aspirin but it didn't seem to make much difference to me.
D: When do they come on?
P: They seem to be there all day long, and at night I just can't get to sleep.
D: So they are bad enough to keep you awake?
P: Yes.
D: And how do you feel in yourself?
P: Very weak, and I'm tired of course. I think I've lost some weight.
D: Have you had headaches in the past?
P: Just one or two, but never anything like this.

Task 4

Results of investigations:

ESR – 80 mm in 1st hour
Neutrophils – 85%
Biopsy showed the changes of giant cell arteritis.

Task 6 and Language focus 2

D: Well Mr Jameson, there's a nerve running behind your knee and your hip and through your spine. When you lift your leg, that nerve should slide in and out your spine quite freely. But with your leg, the nerve won't slide very far. When you lift it, the nerve gets trapped and it's very sore. When I bend your knee, that takes the tension off and eases the pain. If we straighten it, the nerve goes taut and it's painful.

   Now what is trapping the nerve? Well, your X-ray confirms that you've got a damaged disc in the lower part of your back. The disc is a little pad of gristle which lies between the bones in your spine. If you lift heavy loads in the wrong way, you can damage it. And that's what's happened to you. You've damaged a disc. It's pressing on a nerve in your spine so that it can't slide freely and that's the cause of these pains you've been having.

   Now we're going to try to solve the problem first of all with bed rest to let the disc get back to normal and with drugs to take away the pain and help the disc recover. We'll also give you some physio to ease your leg and back. I can't promise this will be entirely successful and we may have to consider an operation at a later date.

Unit 7   Treatment

Task 2

P: Have I got to rest? I was hoping that you could give me something to ease the pain so that I could get back to work.

D: Well I'm afraid going back to work is out of the question just now. I think it will be some weeks before you can go back to your kind of active work. You're going to have to rest and to begin with at least two weeks of complete bed rest. You must rest to allow this swelling to go down and be absorbed to reduce the pressure on the nerve and lessen the pain. Movement will only increase the pressure. If you get up, even to sit on a chair, all the body weight above the damaged disc will press down on the disc below causing more pressure with the risk of pushing out more of the soft disc centre and making the problem worse. Rest also helps to relieve the tight muscle spasm. So for the first week it should be complete bed rest on a firm, hard mattress, a low pillow, better still, no pillow. You should also try to have your meals lying down. Don't sit up to eat. I'll give you drugs to relieve the pain and stiff muscles. When the pain and stiffness improves I'll get the physiotherapist to instruct you in exercises to strengthen your back muscles, and to make you more supple and we'll then gradually mobilise you, letting you get up for longer each day, being guided by the pain you are experiencing.

   So this will have to be the programme. It's not a condition which you can get up and work off, I'm afraid.

Task 6

Physio: First of all you lie down on your tummy on a hard surface. The floor will do. Now place your hands on your back and lift one leg up straight without bending your knee. Then bring it down and lift the other leg up in the same way and then bring it down. Repeat this exercise five times doing it alternately with each leg.

   Keeping the same position, place your hands on your back and lift your chest up off the floor, and then bring it down slowly. Repeat this exercise five times.

   Now keeping your hands at your sides and lying on your tummy, lift alternate leg and arm simultaneously (for example your right leg and left arm), and then bring them down. Next lift your other alternate leg and arm, and then bring them down. Repeat this exercise five times.

   Keep your hands on your back and then lift your chest and legs up simultaneously, and then bring them down slowly. Repeat this exercise also five times. (This is a difficult exercise but with practice you'll be able to do it properly.)

   Now you have to change position. So lie on your back with your hands on your sides and bend your knees up, keeping your feet on the floor. Now lift up your bottom and then bring it down slowly. Repeat this exercise five times.

   You should do these exercises three times a day, preferably on an empty stomach before meals. Then, depending on your progress, after two weeks or so we'll increase the number of times you do these exercises. You should try to do them as slowly and smoothly as possible and try to avoid jerking your body.

Key

Unit 1   Taking a history I

Task 1

SURNAME	Hall		FIRST NAMES	Kevin
AGE 32	SEX M		MARITAL STATUS	M
OCCUPATION	Lorry driver			
PRESENT COMPLAINT		frontal headaches 3/12 worse in a.m. "Dull, throbbing" relieved by lying down also $^c/_o$ deafness		

1 morning
2 complains of
3 male
4 married
5 They are the patient's own words.
6 for three months (similarly 3/52 = three weeks; 3/7 = three days)

Practice 3

Use this diagram to tell you where to indicate in each case.

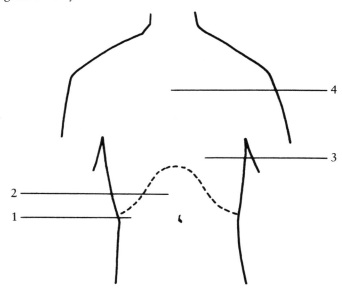

Role-play 1

B: Use this additional information to answer any questions the doctor asks.

1 Greasy food, like fried eggs, upsets you most. The pain lasts several hours.
2 The pain wakes you at night. Usually early in the morning. Spicy food brings on the pain. Too much to drink also makes it worse.
3 The pain is really bad. You've been coughing up brownish spit. You've had a temperature.
4 You've had a cold. You're not coughing up phlegm.

Solutions:

1 gall bladder
2 duodenal ulcer
3 pneumonia
4 tracheitis

Task 2

(A full list of abbreviations is given in Appendix 2.)

O/E on examination
BP blood pressure
CNS central nervous system
-ve negative
? query/possible
1/52 one week

Task 3

1 What's your occupation?
  What do you do?
  What's your job?

2 Whereabouts was the pain?
  Show me where the pain was.

3 When did the pain first happen?

5 Did anything make it better?

6 Does anything special bring it on?

7 Are your parents alive?
  How old was your father when he died?
  What age did your father die at?

Task 4

1 Green
2 42
3 Salesman
4 Central
5 10 mins
6 clear/normal
7 pulse
8 BP
9 HS

Practice 4

a) What's your name?
   How old are you?
   Are you married?
   What's your job?
   What's brought you here today?
   Where exactly is the pain?
   How long have you had it?
   Did anything special bring it on?
   Is it worse at any particular time?
   Does anything make it better or worse?
   Have you any other problems?
   Have you taken anything for it?
   Did the aspirin help?

b) How long have you been suffering from these headaches?
   How long do they last?
   How often do you get them?
   Do they ever make you feel sick?
   Have you noticed any other problems?
   How does the pain affect you?

Task 5

1 63
2 feverish, running nose, aches in muscles, generalised malaise
3 confused and delirious
4 bleeding haemorrhoids
5 white count 21,000/mm^3, 90% lymphocytes
6 chronic lymphatic leukaemia
7 asymptomatic
8 moderate drinker

Task 6

SURNAME Hudson	FIRST NAMES William Henry
AGE 58 SEX M	MARITAL STATUS M
OCCUPATION Postmaster	
PRESENT COMPLAINT ^{c}/o severe low back pain. 1/52 radiating to left leg. Accompanied by parasthesia. Unable to sleep because of pain. Unrelieved by aspirin. May have started after gardening.	

Unit 2   Taking a history II

Task 1

System	Complaint	No complaint	Order
ENT			
RS		✓	3
CVS		✓	4
GIS		✓	1
GUS		✓	2
CNS		✓	5
Psychiatric	✓		6

Practice 1

1 (c), 2 (f), 3 (b), 4 (d), 5 (a), 6 (e).

Role-play 1

Information for **B** (patient):

1 You are a 60-year-old electrician.
You have coughed up blood several times over the last few weeks.
You have noticed that you're losing weight. Your clothes don't fit you properly.
You smoke 30 cigarettes a day.

2 You are 68. You are a retired schoolteacher.
You have been getting more and more constipated over the past few months. You've noticed blood in your stools.
You've been losing weight.

3 You are 45. You are a housewife. You have three children.
You get a pain in your stomach after meals. Sometimes you feel squeamish. Fried and oily foods seem to be worst.

4 You are a 24-year-old typist.
You have pain when you are passing water. There is blood in your water.
You have to pass water more frequently than usual.

5 You are a student of 19.
You have a headache at the front of your head, along the brow.
Your nose keeps running.
Your headache is worse in the morning when you get up.
It also gets worse when you bend down.

Diagnoses

a) cancer of the colon
b) sinusitis
c) cancer of the lung
d) cystitis
e) cholelithiasis

Solutions

See foot of page 109.

Tasks 3 and 4

FEVER	duration	✓ 1	chills			
	frequency		sweats			
	time	✓ 2	night sweats	✓ 3		
			rigor	✓ 4		
GENERAL SYMPTOMS	malaise	✓ 5	wt loss	✓ 7	anorexia	✓ 8
	weakness		drowsiness		vomiting	
	myalgia	✓ 6	delirium		photophobia	
	bleeding?		nose			
			skin			
			urine			
ACHES AND PAINS	head		abdomen		loin	
	teeth		chest		back	
	eyes		neck		pubic	
	muscle					
	joints					
	bone					

SKIN	rash		**CVS**	dyspnoea	c	
	pruritis			palpitations		
	bruising			ht irregularity		
GIS	diarrhoea		**RESPIRATORY**	cough	✓ 9	
	melaena	e		coryza	F	
				sore throat		
				dyspnoea	c	
URINARY	dysuria	a		pleuritic pain	✓ 11	
	frequency			sputum		
	strangury			haemoptysis	✓ 10	
	discolouration					
NEURO-LOGICAL	vision					
	photophobia	d				
	blackouts					
	diplopia	b				

Practice 2

(Other questions are also possible.)

3   Does the pain come on at any particular time?
4   Apart from the pain, do you feel anything else wrong?
5   Do you smoke? How many do you smoke?
6   When did you first notice the pain?
7   Have you noticed any change in the frequency of the pain?
8   How has your weight been?
9   Do you ever become aware of your heart beating too quickly?
10 Have you had any problem with swelling of the ankles?

There are many possible orders for the questions depending on the patient's responses. This could be a point for discussion.

Language focus 2

2 weight
3 cough
4 blood
5 chest

Practice 3

1 (k), 2 (c), 3 (f), 4 (j), 5 (l), 6 (d), 7 (i),
8 (b), 9 (a), 10 (e), 11 (g), 12 (h).

Role-play 3

Name:	Mr Peter Wilson
Age:	48
Sex:	M
Marital status:	M
Occupation:	Steelrope worker

You had an attack of chest pain last night. The pain was behind your breastbone. You also had an aching pain in your neck and right arm. The pain lasted for 15 minutes. You were very restless and couldn't sleep. You've also been coughing up rusty coloured spit.

For the past year you've suffered from breathlessness when you walk uphill or climb stairs. You've had a cough for some years. You often bring up phlegm. In the past three weeks on three occasions you've felt a tight pain in the middle of your chest. The pain spreads to your right arm. These pains happened when you were working in the garden. They lasted a few minutes. Your ankles feel puffy. You find that your shoes feel tight by the evening although this swelling goes away after you've had a night's rest. You've had cramp pains in your right calf for the last month whenever you walk any distance. If you rest, the pains go away.

You've been in good health in the past although you had whooping cough and wheezy bronchitis as a child. You smoke 20 to 30 cigarettes a day. Your mother is still alive, aged 80. Your father died of a heart attack when he was 56. You have one sister. She had TB when she was younger.

Task 5

1 breathlessness
2 productive
3 oedema
4 intermittent claudication
5 retrosternal/central
6 rusty

Solutions to Role-play 1 (page 107)

1 (c), 2 (a), 3 (e), 4 (d), 5 (b).

Task 6

7 short
8 orthopneic
9 cyanosis
10 clubbing
11 regular
12 oedema
13 some
14 venous
15 clavicular
16 heart
17 crepitations
18 right
19 IV
20 IM

Task 7

SURNAME Jameson	**FIRST NAMES** Alan	
AGE 53 **SEX** M	**MARITAL STATUS** M	
OCCUPATION Carpenter		
PRESENT COMPLAINT Acute backache referred down R sciatic nerve distribution. Began 6/52 ago and became more severe over past 2/52. Affecting work and wakening him at night. Also ^{c}/o tingling in R foot. Wt loss 3 kg. Depressed.		

IMMEDIATE PAST HISTORY Paracetamol helped a little with previous intermittent back pain.

Task 8

1 What's
2 when
3 did
4 Was/Is
5 Has
6 had
7 in
8 that/this
9 other
10 with
11 in
12 Did
13 find
14 on

Task 9

(Other answers are possible.)

a) What's brought you here today?
   Where is the pain?
c) Does the pain affect your sleep?
d) Apart from the pain, have you noticed any other problems?
e) Is it affecting your work?
f) Have you noticed any change in your weight?
g) Have you ever had any problem like this before?
h) Did you take anything for it?
   Did it help?

The hospital doctor is probably a neurologist or an orthopaedic surgeon.

Task 10

	Angina	*Pericarditis*
Site	substernal	retrosternal or across the chest
Radiation	both arms especially ulnar aspect of left arm	back and trapezium ridge, either or both arms
Duration	few minutes only	several hours
Precipitating factors	exertion, emotion, unfamiliar tasks, cold air, eating	coughing, inspiration, changes in body position
Relief of pain	rest, few minutes after taking nitro-glycerine	sitting up, leaning forward
Accompanying symptoms	breathlessness	

Task 11

See 3.4

Task 12

On the cassette the doctor does not always speak in sentences. Sometimes he stops in the middle of what he is saying, says 'um' or 'er' and repeats himself. This is typical of spoken language and gives the doctor time to think.

Unit 3   Examining a patient

Task 1

1 (e), 2 (c), 3 (a), 4 (d), 5 (b), 6 (f).

Task 2

1 (d), 2 (b), 3 (e), 4 (a), 5 (c).

Practice 2

(Other answers are possible.)

1 Firstly I'd like you to kneel on that straight-backed chair so that your feet are just slightly hanging over the edge. That's right. Now I'm going to tap them behind your heel with this hammer. This is just a method of testing for your ankle jerk. That's fine.

2 Now I'd like you to sit with your legs just dangling over the edge of the couch so that I can test your knee jerks. Now nothing very much is happening here, so what I'd like you to do is to clasp your hands together with the fingers and try to pull your fingers apart. Pull as hard as you can and concentrate on pulling. That's fine. That makes it a lot easier to produce your knee jerk.

3 Now finally I want you to lie down on the bed with your legs stretched out in front of you. Now I'm going to place my hand on your knee and with this key I'm going to stroke the sole of your foot to see which way your big toe will turn. This is called the plantar reflex. You shouldn't find it painful although it may tickle a little. Fine. Now I'll check the other foot. Very good. That's your reflexes all finished now. Thank you.

Task 3

1	lie	6	press
2	lift/raise	7	hurt
3	bend	8	roll
4	bend	9	feel
5	straighten	10	lift/raise

You can listen to the complete dialogue on your cassette.

Task 4

1 radial pulses
2 BP
3 heart sounds
4 lungs
5 abdomen
6 femoral pulses

Task 5

THE FIRST EXAMINATION

1 Height
2 Weight ✓
3 Auscultation of heart and lungs
4 Examination of breasts and nipples
5 Examination of urine ✓
6 Examination of pelvis
7 Examination of legs ✓
8 Inspection of teeth
9 Estimation of blood pressure ✓
10 Blood sample for blood group
11 Blood sample for haemoglobin
12 Blood sample for serological test for syphilis
13 Blood sample for rubella antibodies
14 Examination of abdomen to assess size of uterus ✓
15 Examination of vagina and cervix

(a) 5, (b) 9, (c) 2, (d) 11, (e) 7, (f) 14.

Task 6

(Suggested order)

1 (a), 2 (c), 3 (f), 4 (e), 5 (b), 6 (d).

Role-play 1

D: How are you, Mrs Wallace?
P: I'm fine.
D: Have you brought your urine sample?
P: Yes, here it is.
D: I'll just check it. Fine, just slip off your coat and I'll check your weight next. Urine is all clear. Your weight is 87.5 kilos. You've gained rather a lot since your last visit. Four kilos. I think you'll have to cut down a bit.
   Now if you'd like to lie down on the couch, I'll take a look at the baby. I'll just measure to see what height it is. Right. The baby seems slightly small. This might be because your dates are wrong. Remember you weren't sure of your last period. The best thing would be to have a scan done. I'll make an appointment for you next week. The baby's in the right position. It's coming head first. Now I'm going to listen for the baby's heartbeat. That's fine. I can hear it quite clearly. Have you noticed any swelling of your ankles?
P: Not really.
D: Let's have a quick look. No, they seem to be all right. Now, would you like to sit up and I'll take your blood pressure? It's quite normal. Now I'll take a sample of blood to check your haemoglobin. Fine. You can get your shoes and coat on again now.

Task 7

1   gentamicin, erythromycin
2   co-trimoxazole, erythromycin
3   ampicillin
4   ampicillin, co-trimoxazole
5   benzylpenicillin
6   gentamicin, benzylpenicillin
7   tetracycline
8   phenoxymethylpenicillin, benzylpenicillin
9   tetracycline
10 erythromycin

Task 8

D: I'll just check a few things to see if we can get to the bottom of these problems. First of all I'll check your pulse and then I'll do your blood pressure. I'd like you to take off your jacket and roll up your sleeve.

P: How is it doctor?

D: It's just a little above normal, but that doesn't mean too much. If you'd like to roll up your shirt, I'm going to check your heart and lungs. Now just breathe normally. Good. Now I'd like you to take deep breaths in and out through your mouth. That's fine. Now if you'd like to lie down on the couch, I'll examine your stomach.

P: Right oh.

D: Take a deep breath in and out. And again. Now I'll just see if there's any sign of a hernia. Could you slip your trousers down? That's fine. Give a cough please. Again please. Now because you've been having trouble with your waterworks, I'd like to examine your back passage. If you'd roll over on to your left side and bend your knees up. You might find this a bit uncomfortable, but it won't take long. That's it. All finished. You can get your clothes on now.

Task 9

> Dear Mr Fielding,
>
> This recently retired postmaster complains of difficulty
> starting to pass urine and increased frequency. He has nocturia x3.
> Rectal examination shows moderate enlargement of the prostate. I also
> discovered that he has atrial fibrillation which is under treatment
> with digoxin 0.25 mg. There is no cardiac enlargement and his BP
> is 160 / 105. This fibrillation is presumably due to ischaemic heart
> disease, but I felt that he would fairly soon require some surgery
> to the prostate and this may become urgent.
>
> Thank you for seeing him.
>
> Yours sincerely,
>
> Dr Peter Watson

Unit 4   Special examinations

Task 1

SURNAME	Priestly		FIRST NAMES	
AGE		SEX M	MARITAL STATUS	
OCCUPATION	Postman			
PRESENT COMPLAINT				

Failing sight. L eye has deteriorated over past year.
Seriously affecting his work. "can't cope".

The patient has been referred to the Ophthalmology Department (the Eye Clinic).

Task 2

a) all
b) can
c) anything
d) that
e) any
f) that
g) that

(d) and (f) refer to lenses.

Task 3

1 up
2 up
3 up
4 down/up

Practice 1

1 (d),   2 (c),   3 (b),   4 (f),   5 (a),   6 (e).

Practice 2

1 limb power
2 lung vital capacity
3 consolidation of the lungs
4 eye movements
5 temperature
6 rectum
7 co-ordination of the right limb
8 throat/tonsils

Role-play 1

Compare your version with the Tapescript for Task 1.

Task 4

RS, GIS, glands, ENT, height and weight.
Paediatric.
The patient is a 4-year-old girl.

Task 5

a)	going	i)	so
b)	called	j)	you're
c)	might	k)	I'll
d)	of	l)	tickly
e)	going	m)	now
f)	then	n)	all
g)	done	o)	isn't
h)	like		

Task 6

For paediatric examination of throat (1), ears (2), chest (3) and back (4) see the Tapescript for Task 4.

5 *foot*
   D: We'll just ask Mummy to take off your shoes and socks so I can have a quick look at your feet. It might be tickly but it won't be sore.

6 *nasal passage*
   D: Can you sit on Mummy's knee? I'm going to have a look at your nose with this little light. You won't feel anything at all. Can you put your head back to help me?

Tasks 7 and 8

Test Question	Order	Patient's Score
1	1	1
2	8	0
3	7	0
4	6	0
5	5	0
6	3	1
7	4	1
8	–	–
9	2	0

Total score 3/8
= severe impairment

Task 9

1 What was the year of your birth?
2 Can you remember that?
3 What was the date?
4 How old will you be now, do you think?
5 Do you know that?
6 Well tell me, is it summer or winter?
7/8 Or do the days not mean a great deal to you now that you're not working?

b) is question 7
c) is question 5
d) is question 4
e) is question 3
f) is question 2

Practice 3

1 What is this place called?
  Where are we now?

2 Which day is it today?
  What day is this?

3 What is this month called?
  What month are we in now?

4 What year are we in?
  What is the year?

5 How old are you?
  What is your age?

6 When were you born?
  What was your year of birth?

7 What is your date of birth?
  What month were you born in?

8 What's the time?
  Can you tell me the time?

9 How many years have you been living here?
  For how long have you stayed here?

Task 10

1 (b), 2 (a), 3 (c), 4 (d).

Language focus 4

Check your answers with the Tapescript.

117

Task 12

1 Title
2 Authors
3 Abstract
4 Introduction
5 Report of case
6 Comment
7 References

Task 13

1 Missing (Title)
2 (e) (Authors)
3 (b) (Abstract)
4 (c) (Introduction)
5 (f) and (g) (Report of case–Figure 1)
6 (a) (Comment)
7 (d) (References)

Task 14

1 The Title – 'Iatrogenic arteriovenous fistula of the internal mammary artery.'
   – 'Transcatheter intravascular coil occlusion.'

2 The first part of the case report

3 Figure 2

Task 15

1 was	11 a	21 was
2 to	12 had	22 had
3 because	13 of	23 but
4 to	14 since	24 were
5 the	15 had	25 were
6 had	16 to	26 at
7 in	17 was	27 in
8 of	18 on	28 was
9 of	19 to	29 in
10 the	20 was	30 were

Task 16

> Dear Dr Watson,
>
> Your patient, Mr Hudson, was admitted as an emergency on 23 February
> with acute retension of urine due to his enlarged prostate for which he was
> awaiting elective surgery.
>
> On admission to the ward he was still in rapid artrial fibrillation and his blood
> pressure was 180/120. The bladder was distended to the umbilicus and p.r. showed
> an enlarged soft prostate. He was sedated and catheterised. Urinalysis showed
> 3+ glucose and GTT showed a diabetic curve. He was therefore started on diet
> and metformin 500 mg t.d.s.
>
> Dr Wilson, our physician, is dealing with the cardiac side of things before we
> go ahead with the operation.
>
> Yours sincerely,

You should add to the Diagnosis section: (3) ? Diabetes.

Unit 5   Investigations

Task 1

2 your left/right side
3 knees
4 down
5 up
6 still

Practice 1

d) 1
c) 2
a) 3
f) 4
g) 5
e) 6
b) 7

Practice 2

1 ECG

D: Your pulse is a bit irregular. I'm not quite certain why this is but I think we'll have to get a tracing of your heartbeat. I want you to strip down to the waist and also take off your shoes and socks. First of all, this is a completely painless procedure. Are you quite comfortable? It's better if you're as relaxed as possible before I start to take the cardiograph. It only takes a few minutes to do the actual test but it takes a bit longer to get you wired up. I'm just putting some cream on your wrists and ankles. That's everything ready. Now just relax as much as you can.

2 Barium meal

D: Good morning Miss Jones. This test is to help me get a picture of the inside of your gullet and your stomach so that we can find out what's causing you these pains there. I want you just to stand here while I give you a cup of liquid to drink. This liquid will show up after you've drunk it and will be able to tell me if you have an ulcer in your stomach or duodenum. I'd like you to drink the liquid now and I'll be taking pictures of it as it goes down. That's fine. Thank you.

3 Crosby capsule

D: Now I'm just going to give you a little jab to help your tummy relax. Just a little prick. OK? That's fine. Good girl. Now I want you to open your mouth for me so that I can pass this little tube down into your tummy. That's fine. Good girl. Nothing to worry about. Head back a little? That's fine. Now can you swallow for me? And again? Good girl. Now I want you to try and keep as still as possible.

4 Ultrasound scan

D: Good morning Mrs Smith. I'd like you to lie down on this table here. I'll just roll up your night-dress. I'm not sure if you've had a scan before, but it's important to have the area over the baby clean. This oil helps to get a contact so that the picture is clear. We'll just rub in the oil a little bit and now I'll put on the equipment. Try and keep as still as you possibly can. That's good. Now if you turn your head to the left, you'll be able to see the scan as I'm taking it. As you see, it's just like a television picture. This black part here is the baby's head and this is the body. As you can see, it's moving around very well. I'm actually taking pictures of it as we go along and after we've finished I'll be able to take measurements from them so we can work out when your baby is due. That's everything finished now.

5 Myelogram

D: We're going to put a little needle in your back. We'll inject some fluid in, put you on to the table there and take some X-ray pictures. These will help us to know exactly where the trouble is. Now roll on to your left side. That's it. I want you to roll up into a little ball, to bring your knees up and tuck your head down. That's fine. Now I'm going to swab your back. You'll feel it a bit cold. Now you'll feel me pressing on your back. All right? Scratch coming up now. Now you'll feel me pressing in. OK. That's fine. I'm just injecting the stuff in. You shouldn't feel it at all. That's it. OK. I'll just take the needle out now. Now just straighten out gently and lie on your front. We'll take the pictures now.

Task 3

Essential	Possibly useful	Not required
ECG chest X-ray urea and electrolytes urinalysis creatinine IVP (IVU)	radioisotope studies serum cholesterol	serum thyroxine barium meal skull X-ray uric acid

Practice 3

a) chest X-ray, bronchoscopy, sputum culture
b) abdominal ultrasonograph, Hb, EUA and D & C
c) serum thyroxine and T_3 resin uptake ratio
d) cholecystogram, abdominal ultrasonograph
e) Normally no investigations are required. In a hospital situation a physician may choose to give throat swab, monospot, viral antibodies, full blood count.
f) tonometry

Role-play 1

1 Mr Gumley

D: Mr Gumley, you'll have to have some investigations done to find out exactly what's causing your problem. Firstly we need to get your chest X-rayed. Then for three mornings running I'd like you to bring to the surgery a sample of the phlegm that you cough up in the morning. We'll be sending that off to the lab for testing to see if you have any particular germs present. Following that, it'll be necessary for you to have a bronchoscopy done. This is an investigation which involves looking down into your lungs through a tube. We'll have to admit you to hospital for the day to do it. It's not a particularly pleasant investigation but you'll be given an anaesthetic spray before the tube is passed down into your lungs. Usually it doesn't take more than a few minutes, but it may last longer if they need to take samples of the tissue in your lungs – maybe up to 20 minutes. You have to take this test with an empty stomach, so you won't have any breakfast that day. You'll be able to get home again after the test, but you'll have to wait until the anaesthetic has worn off before you eat anything.

2 Mrs Emma Sharp

D: Because of your heavy periods, Mrs Sharp, we must find out if you have become anaemic so I will have to take a blood test. I think it will also be necessary for you to have a D & C done in hospital. We can probably do this as a day case. It is a very simple procedure and just involves removing a small piece of the lining from inside the womb to find out why your periods have become so heavy. It will also give us a better chance to examine you when you are under the anaesthetic. It might also be necessary to do an abdominal ultrasonograph. This is a very simple test which takes a special picture of the lower end of your abdomen to see if the womb is enlarged.

3 Miss Grace Donaldson

D: From your symptoms it would seem that you have an overactive thyroid gland. We can test this quite simply by doing a blood test to check the level of hormones in your blood.

4 *Mr Pritt*

D: Because you have been having this trouble with abdominal pain after fatty foods I think you may have some stones in your gall bladder. You will need to have a special X-ray done. This is called a cholecystogram and it will involve you taking some tablets before attending the X-ray department. They'll take an ordinary X-ray first and then give you something fatty to eat, after which they'll take pictures of the gall bladder area to see if your gall bladder is working properly and if there are any stones present. They may also do an ultrasonograph. This is a way of examining your abdomen using a special machine which can show us pictures of your stomach and gall bladder using sound signals. It's not painful at all and it doesn't take more than five or ten minutes to perform.

5 *Barry Scott*

D: Mrs Scott, I feel certain that Barry has German measles. Sometimes we do a blood test to prove this definitely, but because he is only two and a half I am sure he wouldn't like to have a blood test done, and it would be safer to do nothing.

6 *Mrs Mary Lock*

D: Mrs Lock, I think it's possible that you have a condition called glaucoma which is caused by increased pressure inside the eye. In order to prove this it will be necessary for you to have the pressure inside your eyes measured. We use a small instrument with a scale on it to measure the pressure. We'll put a few drops of local anaesthetic on your eye so you shouldn't feel anything. The test only takes a few seconds.

Task 4

**TELEPHONE REPORT FROM
HAEMATOLOGY LABORATORY**

PATIENTS NAME   UNIT NO

HALL Kevin

	BLOOD FILM
WBC x10^9/L 7.2	NEUTRO .... 60 %
Hb g/dl 12.9	LYMPH .... 30 %
Hct 0.39	MONO .... 5 %
MCVfl 81	EOSINO .... 4 %
Platelets x10^9/L 264	BASO .... 1 %
ESR mm 43	

OTHER INFORMATION

.... RBC 3.32 ....

.... burr cells ++ ....

....

PROTHROMBIN RATIO .... :1

TIME MESSAGE RECEIVED .... AM/PM

MESSAGE RECEIVED BY ....

DATE RECEIVED ....

Task 5

(Other answers are possible.)

Sodium is elevated.
Potassium is raised.
Bicarbonate is low.
Plasma urea is abnormally high.

Task 6

1 complained	8 12.9
2 found	9 43 mm
3 normal	10 burr
4 blocker	11 greatly/very
5 diuretic	12 50.1
6 elevated/high/raised	13 16
7 albumen	14 chronic renal failure

Task 7

Dear Dr Jones

Thank you for referring this pleasant 42-year-old salesman. These episodes of central chest pain which he describes with radiation to the L arm and fingers sound very typical of angina. Physical examination was unrevealing.

I have checked various blood parameters including serum cholesterol and total glycerol. CXR was normal but exercise ECG showed ST depression.

Serum cholesterol was elevated at 7.2 mmol/l.

I will be seeing him again next week to let him have these results. I shall arrange for him to be seen by the dietician and prescribe bezafibrate 600 mg daily. In view of the family history I am sure this will be worthwhile.

Yours sincerely,

Paul Scott

Dr Paul Scott

Task 8

1 Title
2 Authors
3 Abstract
4 Introduction
5 Patients and methods
6 Results
7 Discussion
8 Acknowledgements
9 References

Task 9

1 Title
2 Abstract
3 Final paragraph of discussion
4 Interesting diagrams/tables
5 Introduction
6 Authors
7 References
8 Patients and methods (– if you were interested in carrying out a similar experiment.)

Task 10

1 were	9 for	17 out
2 for	10 to	18 who
3 Their	11 and	19 of
4 from	12 were	20 of
5 to	13 out	21 of
6 though	14 out	22 is
7 of	15 which	23 were
8 The	16 by	24 out

Task 11   *William Hudson*

1 diarrhoea
2 metformin (Glucophage)
3 three
4 cardiac
5 dehydrated
6 semi-comatose
7 irregular
8 abdomen
9 tenderness
10 absent
11 possible
12 TUR – transurethral resection

Role-play 2

A (Consultant)

Your father's condition is quite poor. It seems that he's had diarrhoea for six days and this may have affected his diabetes. As you know, any infection can cause diabetes to get out of control. He's very dehydrated and so the first thing we'll be doing is giving him some fluid. We'll also check his blood sugar and he'll have an X-ray done of his chest and abdomen. Lastly we'll be checking to see which particular germ caused his diarrhoea.

The investigations are:

X-ray chest/abdomen;
blood urea and electrolytes;
blood sugar;
stool culture.

Unit 6   Making a diagnosis

Task 1

SURNAME Nicol	FIRST NAMES Harvey
AGE 59 SEX M	MARITAL STATUS M
OCCUPATION Office worker	

PRESENT COMPLAINT
   ^c/o headaches, L side for 3/52, unrelieved by aspirin.
   Initially flu - like symptoms. Unable to sleep.
   Slight weight loss. Feels "weak and tired".	

Task 2

(Other answers are possible.)

space-occupying lesion
migraine
viral fever
aneurism
temporal arteritis
depression
cervical spondylosis

Task 3

temporal arteritis
migraine
depression

unlikely – space-occupying lesion, viral fever, aneurism
excluded – cervical spondylosis
Investigations – full blood count and ESR
 – skull X-ray
 – superficial left temporal artery biopsy

Task 4

Raised ESR and polymorphs strongly indicate and the biopsy confirms that the patient
 has temporal cell arteritis.
Normal skull X-ray excludes space-occupying lesion.

Practice 1

1 nephrotic syndrome
2 Henoch-Schonlein syndrome
3 mononucleosis, glandular fever
4 cholelithiasis
5 scleroderma

Task 6

1 explanation of cause
2 proposed treatment
3 warning of possible operation

Practice 2

1 The pancreas is a gland near the stomach which helps digestion and also makes insulin.
2 The thyroid is a gland in the neck which controls the rate at which your body works.
3 Fibroids are growths in the womb which are not cancerous but cause heavy bleeding.
4 Emphysema is a condition in which the structure of the lung is destroyed and makes
 breathing difficult.
5 An arrhythmia is an irregularity of the heartbeat, for example when you have an
 extra beat.
6 Bone marrow is where the various types of blood cells are made.
7 The prostate gland produces some of the secretions which mix with semen. Sometimes
 it becomes enlarged and causes trouble in passing water.
8 This is what happens when acid from your stomach comes back up into the gullet.
 It causes heartburn.

Practice 3

1 It may cause stomach pain.
2 The baby may be born with deformities.
3 You may burst a blood vessel in the gullet.
4 You can develop dermatitis.
5 You may have a stroke.
6 He will get diarrhoea.
7 You may have a heart attack.
8 It may develop changes of arthritis.

Role-play 1

See Key, Unit 7, Practice 1.

Task 7

1 Title – 'Practice of preoperative assessment by anaesthetists'
2 Abstract (a)
3 Final paragraph of Discussion (b)
4 Interesting tables (c)
5 Introduction (d)
6 Authors (e)
7 References (f)

Task 8

1 was	13 in	25 was
2 in	14 before	26 to
3 to	15 Each	27 for
4 as	16 for	28 those
5 they	17 of	29 which
6 of	18 in	30 with
7 of	19 of	31 that
8 They	20 which	32 were
9 about	21 of	33 with
10 of	22 to	34 with
11 of	23 them	35 were
12 This	24 which	36 to

Role-play 2

A (Surgeon)

We've operated on your father and discovered that he'd had a blockage of the blood supply to his small bowel. This caused the small bowel to become gangrenous and it had to be removed. He'll be able to manage without it but it is a fairly major operation and naturally his condition is serious. The blockage of blood supply caused his diarrhoea, and because of the diarrhoea his diabetes went out of control as he lost so much fluid and salts from his body. That explains why he went into a coma.

Unit 7   Treatment

Tasks 1 and 2

SURNAME Jameson	**FIRST NAMES** Alan	
AGE 53 **SEX** M	**MARiTAL STATUS** M	

OCCUPATION   Carpenter

PRESENT COMPLAINT   Acute backache referred down R sciatic nerve
distribution. Began 6/52 ago and became more severe over past 2/52.
Affecting work and wakening him at night. Also ^{c}/o tingling in
R foot. Wt loss 3 kg. Depressed.

O/E
General Condition   Fit, well - muscled.

ENT   NAD

RS   NAD

CVS   Normal pulsations at femoral popliteal,
posterior tibial + dorsalis pedis.

GIS   NAD

GUS   NAD

CNS   Loss of lumbar lordosis, spasm of R erector spinal.
Straight leg raising R restricted to 45°.
Reflexes present & equal. Neurol - depressed R ankle jerk.

IMMEDIATE PAST HISTORY
Paracetamol helped a little with previous intermittent back pain.

POINTS OF NOTE
Carpenter - active work
1.78 m, 68 kg - tall, slightly-built

INVESTIGATIONS   X-ray - narrowing of disc space between
lumbar 4 & 5. Myelogram - posterior lateral herniation of disc.

DIAGNOSIS
Prolapsed intervertebral disc.

MANAGEMENT
dihydrocodeine   2 q.d.s p.c.
Physio

Practice 1

1 *A hypertensive 50-year-old director of a small company*

D: The condition you have requires to be controlled to prevent future damage to the body, especially the blood vessels. If it is not controlled you can have certain serious illnesses such as a heart attack or a stroke. Treatment is therefore to prevent illness developing because I am sure that you do not feel ill at the moment. You will have to take tablets, or medicine, but will also have to modify some of your habits, for instance, you must stop smoking.

2 *An insulin-dependent 11-year-old girl accompanied by her mother*

D: Now Elizabeth, the trouble with you is that you are not making a substance that you need to control the amount of sugar in your blood. If you have too much sugar or too little sugar it will make you feel very ill and we will have to replace this each day. It means that you will have to have a jab because it doesn't work properly if we give it to you in a tablet. Your mother, here, will go with you to see the nurse and she will show you how to do it. Many other boys and girls, some much younger than you, soon learn to do it, so you don't need to be frightened.

3 *A 65-year-old schoolteacher with osteoarthritis of the left hip*

D: This condition is really like the wear and tear of a hinge. The joint is becoming stiff and painful because it is roughened by inflammation. Fortunately, as you are now retired, you will be able to modify your life so that it does not trouble you so much. I will prescribe tablets which will help the pain and stiffness and, although this will not cure it, it will control the discomfort. If, in the future, it gets more troublesome we can always consider an operation which will get rid of the pain.

4 *A 23-year-old lorry driver affected by epilepsy*

D: Unfortunately, the attacks which you have been having are shown to be quite severe. They are caused by abnormal electrical activity in your brain. This is called epilepsy. But we can help to stop you having fits. I will prescribe tablets for you which will control the condition as long as you are taking them. It is most important that you take them regularly and don't forget. The problem as far as you are concerned, is that you are not permitted to drive for at least three years after your last attack. It will perhaps be necessary for you to consider changing your occupation, so you must inform your employer of this in the first place.

5 *A 52-year-old cook with carcinoma of the bowel*

D: The tests show that you have got a nasty growth in the bowel which will have to be removed. It is far too dangerous to leave it. The operation has every chance of removing the disease. The exact type of operation, however, will depend upon what the surgeon finds at operation, but the possibility is that you may have to have an opening made on the skin of your abdomen. This is something which a lot of people can cope with and may only be of a temporary nature.

6 *A 27-year-old teacher of handicapped children suffering from a depressive illness*

D: I know that you feel that this illness is something which you feel is affecting your whole life. It is called depression and is thought to be due to chemical changes in the brain. It's not something you can pull yourself out of – you will need help in the way of psychotherapy and drugs as well. You may think that nobody else has ever felt like you are feeling before, but let me assure you that this is quite a common condition and that you will get well again, although it will take some weeks before you feel improved. Often it is possible to continue in your routine of work because this gives you something rewarding to do while you are getting better. You will get a medicine to take which will take some weeks to work, so don't be more despondent, if at first it does not seem to be helping.

7 A 6-month-old baby boy suffering from atopic eczema, accompanied by his mother

D: This skin condition which your baby has is not an infection and so he cannot give the condition to anybody. It is a condition which is affecting the skin and will require ointments from time to time and will vary according to circumstances but sometimes it will seem better and then it will flare up again. This condition is really a constitutional one and so heredity factors from yourself or your husband have a part to play in causing it.

Task 3

a) 6 hrly
b) for pain
c) 100 tablets
d) dihydrocodeine BP
e) give
f) write/put
g) after food/meals
h) tablets

Task 4

1   tablets
2   two
3   six
4/5 after food/meals
6   can
7   pain

You can listen to the doctor's instructions on your cassette.

Task 5

1 Patient (c)
2 Patient (f)
3 Patient (e)
4 Patient (b)
5 Patient (a)
6 Patient (g)
7 Patient (d)

a) twice a day
b) three times a day

Task 6

1 (d)
2 (b)
3 (e)
4 (c)
5 (a)

Practice 3

1 You should lie on a hard surface.
2 You should be careful while getting out of bed. Try to roll over and then get up from your side.
3 You should (try to) avoid bending forward, for example, if you are picking up something off the floor.
4 You should try to bend your knees and keep your back straight.
5 You should (try to) avoid lifting heavy weights.

Practice 5

D: Well, Mr Jameson, I am sorry to see that your back is still causing you pain and that you have now developed a weakness in your right foot. The weakness is due to the continued pressure on the nerve roots supplying the muscles of your leg. This pressure, of course, is taking place at the level of the disc between the lumbar vertebrae. Due to this worsening of the condition I think that there is now a strong possibility that you require an operation on the back to remove the disc where it's pressing on the nerve. The operation will need to be carried out by a surgeon specialised in this work, a neurosurgeon. The operation itself will only immobilise you for a few days and you'll soon be up and about again and back to the physiotherapist to improve the strength of your muscles, both in your back and this leg. If you don't have the operation, the risk is that your right foot will be permanently weak. We want to avoid this at all costs. Are there any questions you would like to ask me?

Task 7

Sheet No. ......1...... ...... *Please use a ball point pen*

PRESCRIPTION SHEET

PLEASE ✓ WHEN MEDICINES ARE PRESCRIBED ON

Fluid (Additive Medicine) Prescription Chart	
Diabetic Chart	
Anticoagulant Chart	
Anaesthetic Prescription Sheet	
Record of Labour Sheet	

If medicine discontinued because of suspected adverse reaction please enter in box below

	MEDICINE	ADVERSE REACTION
1		
2		

DIET

Date	DETAILS	Initials

ORAL and OTHER NON-PARENTERAL MEDICINES – REGULAR PRESCRIPTIONS

CODE	Date Commenced	MEDICINES (Block Letters)	DOSE	Method of Admin.	AM 6	AM 8	AM 10	MD 12	PM 2	PM 6	PM 10	MN 12	Other Times	DOCTOR'S SIGNATURE	Discontinued Date	Discontinued Initials
A	15/9/85	ASPIRIN	300 mg	p.o.	X											
B	"	PARACETAMOL	1g	p.o.	X		X		X	X						
C	"	TEMAZEPAM	20 mg	p.o.							X					
D	"	ATENOLOL	100 mg	p.o.	X											
E	"	ISOSORBIDE MONONITRATE	40 mg	p.o.	X					X						
F	"	THYROXINE	0.1 mg	p.o.		X										
G	"	NIFEDIPINE	20 mg	p.o.	X				X		X					
H	"	GTN TRANSDERMAL PATCH	5 mg	patch	X											
I	"	BENDROFLUAZIDE /	1 tab	p.o.		X										
J		POTASSIUM CHLORIDE														
K																
L																

PARENTERAL MEDICINES – REGULAR PRESCRIPTIONS

CODE	Date Commenced	MEDICINE	DOSE	Method of Admin.	AM 6	AM 8	AM 10	MD 12	PM 2	PM 6	PM 10	MN 12	Other Times	DOCTOR'S SIGNATURE	Discontinued Date	Discontinued Initials
M	"	SODIUM HEPARIN	5000u	s.c.	X				X	X						
N	"	DIAMORPHINE	5 mg	IM									4 hrly p.r.n.			
O	"	CYCLIZINE	50 mg	IM									4 hrly p.r.n.			
P	"	GTN	600µg	s.l.									p.r.n.			
Q																

ORAL and OTHER NON-PARENTERAL MEDICINES – ONCE ONLY PRESCRIPTIONS

Date	MEDICINE	DOSE	Method of Admin.	Time of Admin.*	Given by Initials	Time if Diff.*	DOCTOR'S SIGNATURE

PARENTERAL MEDICINES – ONCE ONLY PRESCRIPTIONS

Date	MEDICINE	DOSE	Method of Admin.	Time of Admin.*	Given by Initials	Time if Diff.*	DOCTOR'S SIGNATURE

NAME OF PATIENT	AGE	UNIT NUMBER	CONSULTANT
WYNNE, John	58	1563526	MR SWAN

KNOWN DRUG/MEDICINE SENSITIVITY

Tasks 8 and 9

Discharge Summary (Page 2)

OPERATION: CAVG x4, single saphenous grafts to LAD and RCA,
             sequential saphenous graft to OM1 and OM2.

SURGEON: A. Swan   Assistant: Mr Dickson   GA: Dr Wood

INCISIONS: Median sternotomy and right thigh and leg.

FINDINGS: Dense inferior left ventricular scarring, less marked
             scarring of inferior right ventricle. Fair overall left
ventricular contraction. Diffuse coronary artery disease. All vessels
measuring about 1.5 mm in diameter.

PUMP PERFUSION DATA: Membrane oxygenator, linear flow, aortic SVC
                       and IVC cannulae, LV apical vent. Whole body
cooling to 28°C, cold cardioplegic arrest and topical cardiac
hypothermia for the duration of the aortic cross clamp. Aortic cross
clamp time 54 minutes, total bypass time 103 minutes.

PROCEDURE: Vein was prepared for use as grafts. Systemic heparin
             was administered and bypass established, the left ventricle
was vented, the aorta was cross-clamped and cold cardioplegic arrest
of the heart obtained. Topical cooling was continued for the duration
of the aortic cross clamp.
   Attention was first turned to the first and second obtuse marginal
branches of the circumflex coronary artery. The first obtuse marginal
was intramuscular with proximal artheroma. It admitted 1.5 mm occluder
and was grafted with saphenous sequential grafts, side to side using
continuous 6/0 special prolene which was used for all subsequent
distal anastomoses. The end of this saphenous graft was recurved
and anastomosed to the second obtuse marginal around a 1.75 mm occluder.
   The left anterior descending was opened in its distal half and
accepted a 1.5 mm occluder around which it was grafted with a single
length of long saphenous vein.
   Lastly, the right coronary artery was opened at the crux and again
grafted with a single length of saphenous vein around a 1.5 mm occluder
whilst the circulation was rewarmed.
   The aortic cross clamp was released and air vented from the left
heart and ascending aorta. Proximal vein anastomoses to the ascending
aorta were completed using continuous 5/0 prolene. The heart was
defibrillated into sinus rhythm with a single counter shock and weaned
off bypass with minimal adrenalin support. Protamine sulphate was
administered and blood volume was adjusted. Cannulae were removed and
cannulation and vent sites repaired. Haemostasis was ascertained.
Pericardial and mediastinal argyle drains were inserted.

CLOSURE: Routine layered closure with ethibond to sternum, dexon
             to presternal and subcutaneous tissues, subcuticular
             dexon to skin.

A. Swan

Task 10

1 cardiac artery venous graft
2 left anterior descending
3 right coronary artery
4 first obtuse marginal
5 left ventricle/ventricular

Task 11

D: The diameter of one of your coronary arteries is reduced so one part of your heart muscle is starved of oxygen and other nutrients. If you don't have an operation, you will continue to have pain in your chest and you may even have a further heart attack. Before serious damage is done, we must try to improve the flow of blood to the heart. We're going to remove a vein from your leg and use it to replace part of your coronary artery. The chances of recovery are very good, and I'm confident you'll feel a lot more comfortable after the operation.

Task 12

– A weekly magazine that gives the contents pages of leading scientific journals.
– Published in the USA by the Institute for Scientific Information Inc.
– Weekly.
– Dependent on country – see section on how to order.

Task 13

Possible answers:

The British Medical Journal 178/179
The Lancet 173/174
Nephron 208
Transplantation 133

Task 14

CC Pg = Current Contents Page   J Pg = Journal Page

Task 15

Ref: Renal transplant/Renal transplantation
CC Pg 133 – *Transplantation* J Pg 461, 467, 471, 529
CC Pg 178 – *The British Medical Journal* J Pg 1477
CC Pg 208 – *Nephron* J Pg 186, 203
CC Pg 173 – *The Lancet* J Pg 1185

Task 16

CC Pg 133

Task 17

(461) 'The clinical and pathological course of hepatitis B liver disease in renal transplant recipients.'
(467) 'The late adverse effect of splenectomy on patient survival following cadaveric renal transplantation.'
(471) 'Excretion of urokallikrein in renal transplant patients.'
(529) 'ABO-autoimmune hemolytic anemia in a renal transplant patient treated with cyclosporine.'

Task 18

1 'The late adverse effect of splenectomy on patient survival following cadaveric renal transplantation.' (467)
2 A distractor – from another journal.*
3 'Specificity of transplantation heterophile antibodies.' (475)
4 'Excretion of urokallikrein in renal transplant patients.' (471)

* From *Nephron* 37: 186–189 (1984) 'Non-typhoid salmonella infections after renal transplantation.'

Appendix 1   Language functions

Casetaking

General information / Personal details

What's your name?
How old are you?
What's your job?
Where do you live?
Are you married?
Do you smoke?
How many do you smoke each day?
Do you drink?
Beer, wine or spirits? (UK)
Beer, wine or alcohol? (US)

Present illness

Starting the interview

What's brought you along today?
What can I do for you?
What seems to be the problem?
How can I help?

Asking about duration

How long have they / has it been bothering you?
How long have you had them/it?
When did they/it start?

Asking about location

Where does it hurt?
Where is it sore?
Show me where the problem is.
Which part of your (head) is affected?
Does it stay in one place or does it go anywhere else?

Asking about type of pain / severity of problem

What's the pain like?
What kind of pain is it?
Can you describe the pain?
Is it bad enough to (wake you up)?
Does it affect your work?
Is it continuous or does it come and go?
How long does it last?

Asking about relieving/aggravating factors

Is there anything that makes it better/worse?
Does anything make it better/worse?

Asking about precipitating factors

What seems to bring it on?
Does it come on at any particular time?

Asking about medication

Have you taken anything for it?
Did (the tablets) help?

Asking about other symptoms

Apart from your (headaches) are there any other problems?

Previous health / Past history

How have you been keeping up to now?
Have you ever been admitted to hospital?
Have you ever had (headaches) before?
Has there been any change in your health since your last visit?

Family history

Are your parents alive and well?
What did he/she die of?
How old was he/she?
Does anyone else in your family suffer from this problem?

Asking about systems

Have you any trouble with (passing water)?
Any problems with (your chest)?
What's (your appetite) like?
Have you noticed any (blood in your stools)?
Do you ever suffer from (headaches)?
Do (bright lights) bother you?
Have you (a spit)?

To rephrase if the patient does not understand, try another way of expressing the same function, for example:

What caused this?
What brought this on?
Was it something you tried to lift?

Examination

Preparing the patient

I'm just going to (test your reflexes).
I'd just like to (examine your mouth).
Now I'm going to (tap your arm).
I'll just check your (blood pressure).

Instructing the patient

Would you (strip to the waist) please?
Can you (put your hands on your hips)?
Could you (bend down and touch your toes)?
Now I just want to see you (walking).
Lift it up as far as you can go, will you?
Let me see you (standing).

Checking if information is accurate

That's tender?

Down here?

The back of your leg?

Commenting/reassuring

I'm checking your (heart) now.
That's fine.
OK, we've finished now.

Confirming information you know

That's tender.

Down here.

The back of your leg.

Investigations

Explaining purpose

I'm going to (take a sample of your bone marrow) to find out what's causing (your anaemia).

Reassuring

It won't take long.
It won't be sore.
I'll be as quick as I can.

Warning

You may feel (a bit uncomfortable).
You'll feel a (jab).

Discussing investigations

Essential	Possibly useful	Not required

should
must
be + required
    essential
    important
    indicated
	could	need not
		
		be + not necessary
		      required
		      important

Essential not to do		
should not must not be + contraindicated		

Making a diagnosis

Discussing certainty

	Certain	Fairly certain	Uncertain
Yes	is must	seems probably likely	might could may
No	can't definitely not exclude rule out	unlikely	possibly a possibility

Explaining the diagnosis

Simple definition

The (disc) is a (little pad of gristle between the bones in your back).

Cause and effect

If we bend the knee, tension is taken off the nerve.
When we straighten it, the nerve goes taut.

Treatment

Advising

I *advise* you to give up smoking.
You'll *have to* cut down on fatty foods.
You *must* rest.
You *should* sleep on a hard mattress.
If you *get up*, all your weight *will* press down on the disc.
Don't sit up to eat.

Expressing regret

I'm afraid that (the operation has not been successful).
I'm sorry to have to tell you that (your father has little chance of recovery).

Appendix 2 Common medical abbreviations

AB	apex beat
abdo.	abdomen
abdms (M)(t)(o)	abdomen without masses, tenderness, organomegaly (US)
a.c.	before meals
ACTH	adrenocorticotrophic hormone
AF	atrial fibrillation
AFP	alphafoetoprotein
A:G	albumin globulin ratio
AHA	Area Health Authority (UK)
AI	aortic incompetence
AJ	ankle jerk
a.m.	morning
AN	antenatal
AP	antero-posterior
APH	antepartum haemorrhage
ARM	artificial rupture of membranes
AS	alimentary system
ASD	atrial septal defect
ASHD	arteriosclerotic heart disease (US)
ASO	antistreptolysin O
ATS	antitetanic serum
A & W	alive and well
AMA	American Medical Association
BB	bed bath; blanket bath
BC	bone conduction
b.d.	twice a day
BF	breast fed
BI	bone injury
BID	brought in dead
b.i.d.	twice a day
BIPP	bismuth iodoform and paraffin paste
BM	bowel movement
BMA	British Medical Association
BMR	basal metabolic rate
BNF	British National Formulary
BNO	bowels not opened
BO	bowels opened
BP	blood pressure
BPC	British Pharmaceutical Codex
BPD	bi-parietal diameter
BS	breath sounds
BUN	blood urea nitrogen (US)
BWt	birth weight

c̄	with
C	head presentation
Ca.	cancer, carcinoma
CAD	coronary artery disease
Capt.	head presentation
CAT	coaxial or computerised axial tomography
CAVG	coronary artery venous graft
CBC	complete blood count (US)
CCF	congestive cardiac failure (UK)
Chr.CF	chronic cardiac failure
Cf.	first certificate (UK)
CF	final certificate (UK)
CFT	complement fixation test
CHF	chronic heart failure; congestive heart failure (US)
CNS	central nervous system
CO	casualty officer (UK)
c/o	complains of
COAD	chronic obstructive airways disease (UK)
COP	change of plaster
COPD	chronic obstructive pulmonary disease (US)
creps	crepitations (UK) (râles US)
C-section	cesarean section (US)
CSF	cerebrospinal fluid
CSSD	Central Sterile Supply Depot (UK)
CSU	catheter specimen of urine
CT	cerebral tumour; coronary thrombosis
CV	cardiovascular
CVA	cardiovascular accident; cerebrovascular accident
CVS	cardiovascular system; cerebrovascular system
Cx	cervix
CXR	chest X-ray
D	divorced
D & C	dilatation and curettage
DD	dangerous drugs
DDA	Dangerous Drugs Act (UK)
decub.	lying down
DHSS	Department of Health and Social Security (UK)
DIC	drunk in charge
dl	decilitre
DN	District Nurse (UK)
DNA	did not attend
DOA	dead on arrival
DRO	Disablement Resettlement Office (UK)
DS	disseminated sclerosis
DTs	delirium tremens
DU	duodenal ulcer
DVT	deep venous thrombosis
D & V	diarrhoea and vomiting
△	diagnosis

E	electrolytes
ECF	extracellular fluid
ECG/EKG(US)	electrocardiogram
ECT	electroconvulsive therapy
EDC	expected date of confinement
EDD	expected date of delivery
EDM	early diastolic murmur
EEG	electroencephalogram
ENT	ear, nose and throat
ESN	educationally sub-normal
ESR	erythrocyte sedimentation rate
ETT	exercise tolerance test
EUA	examination under anaesthesia
F	female
fb	finger breadth
FB	foreign body
FBC	full blood count (UK)
FH	foetal heart
FHH	foetal heart heard
FHNH	foetal heart not heard
fl	femtolitre
FMFF	**foetal movement first felt**
FPC	family planning clinic (UK)
FTBD	fit to be detained; full term born dead
FTAT	**fluorescent treponemal antibody test**
FTND	**full term normal delivery**
FUO	fever of unknown origin
g	gram
GA	general anaesthetic
GB	gall bladder
GC	general condition
GCFT	gonococcal complement fixation test
GI	gastro-intestinal
GOT	glumatic oxaloacetic transaminase
GP	General Practitioner (UK)
GPI	general paralysis of the insane
GPT	glutamic pyruvic transaminase
GTN	glyceryl trinitrate
GTT	glucose tolerance test
GU	gastric ulcer
GUS	genito-urinary system
Gyn.	gynaecology
Hb/Hgb	haemoglobin
HBP	high blood pressure
Hct	haematocrit
H & P	history and physical examination
HP	house physician (UK)
HR	heart rate
HS	**heart sounds**

ICF	intracellular fluid
ICS	intercostal space
ID	infectious disease
IM	intramuscular
IOFB	intra-ocular foreign body
IP	in-patient: interphalangeal
IQ	intelligence quotient
ISQ	in statu quo
IU	international unit
IV	intravenous
IVC	inferior vena cava
IVP	intravenous pyelogram
IVU	intravenous urogram
IZS	insulin zinc suspension
JVD	jugular venous distention (US)
JVP	jugular venous pressure (UK)
KUB	kidney, ureter and bladder
L	left
LA	left atrium; local anaesthetic
LAD	left axis deviation
LBP	low back pain; low blood pressure
LDH	lactic dehydrogenase
LE cells	lupus erythematosus cells
LFTS	lung function tests
LHA	Local Health Authority (UK)
LIF	left iliac fossa
LIH	left inguinal hernia
LKS	liver, kidney and spleen
LLL	left lower lobe
LLQ	left lower quadrant
LMN	lower motor neurone
LMP	last menstrual period; left mento-posterior position of foetus
LOA	left occipito-anterior position of foetus
LOP	left occipito-posterior position of foetus
LP	lumbar puncture
LSCS	lower segment Caesarean section
LUA	left upper arm
LUQ	left upper quadrant
LV	left ventricle: lumbar vertebra
LVE	left ventricular enlargement
LVF	left ventricular failure
LVH	left ventricular hypertrophy
M	male
M/F; M/W/S	male/female; married/widow(er)/single
MCD	mean corpuscular diameter
MCH	mean corpuscular haemoglobin
MCHC	mean corpuscular haemoglobin concentration
MCL	mid-clavicular line
MCV	mean corpuscular volume
MD	mentally deficient

MDM	mid-diastolic murmur
mg	milligram
MI	mitral incompetence insufficiency; myocardial infarction
ml	millilitre
MMR	mass miniature radiography
MO	Medical Officer (UK)
MOH	Medical Officer of Health (UK)
MOP	medical out-patient
MPNI	Ministry of Pensions and National Insurance (UK)
MRC	Medical Research Council (UK)
MS	mitral stenosis; multiple sclerosis; musculo skeletal
MSU	mid-stream urine
MSSU	mid-stream specimen of urine
MSW	Medical Social Worker (UK)
MVP	mitral valve prolapse
NA	not applicable
NAD	no abnormality detected
NBI	no bone injury
ND	normal delivery
NE	not engaged
NIC	National Insurance Certificate (UK)
NND	neo-natal death
nocte	at night
NP	not palpable
NPU	not passed urine
NS	nervous system
NSA	no significant abnormality
NSPCC	National Society for the Prevention of Cruelty to Children (UK)
NYD	not yet diagnosed
OA	on admission; osteo-arthritis
OAP	old age pensioner
OBS	organic brain syndrome
O/E	on examination
oed.	oedema
OM	otitis media
OR	operating room (US)
OT	operating theatre (UK)
P	pulse/protein
Para. 2 + 1	full term pregnancies 2, abortions 1
PAT	paroxysmal atrial tachycardia
PBI	protein bound iodine
p.c.	after food
PDA	patent ductus arteriosus
PERLA	pupils equal and reactive to light and accommodation
PET	pre-eclamptic toxaemia
PID	prolapsed intervertebral disc, pelvic inflammatory disease
Pl.	plasma
p.m.	afternoon
PM	postmortem
PMB	postmenopausal bleeding
PN	postnatal

PND	postnatal depression; paroxysmal nocturnal dyspnoea
PO₂	pressure of oxygen
p.o.	by mouth
POP	plaster of Paris
PPH	postpartum haemorrhage
p.r.	per rectum
p.r.n.	as required
PROM	premature rupture of membranes
PSW	Psychiatric Social Worker (UK)
PU	passed urine; peptic ulcer
PUO	pyrexia of unknown or uncertain origin
p.v.	per vaginam
PVT	paroxysmal ventricular tachycardia
PZI	protamine zinc insulin
q.d.s./q.i.d.	four times a day
R	right; respiration; red
℞	take (used in prescriptions)
RA	rheumatoid arthritis; right atrium
RAD	right axis deviation
RBC	red blood cell count; red blood corpuscles
RBS	random blood sugar
RCA	right coronary artery
Rh.	Rhesus factor; rheumatism
ref.	refer
reg.	regular
RHA	Regional Health Authority (UK)
RI	respiratory infection
RIF	right iliac fossa
RIH	right inguinal hernia
RLL	right lower lobe
RLQ	right lower quadrant
RMO	Regional or Resident Medical Officer (UK)
ROA	right occipital anterior
ROM	range of motion
ROP	right occipital posterior
RS	respiratory system
RTA	road traffic accident
RTC	return to clinic
RUA	right upper arm
RUQ	right upper quadrant
RTI	respiratory tract infection
RVE	right ventricular enlargement
RVH	right ventricular hypertrophy
S	single/sugar
SAH	subarachnoidal haemorrhage
SB	still-born
SBE	sub-acute bacterial endocarditis
s.c.	subcutaneous
SEN	State Enrolled Nurse (UK)
sep.	separated

SG	specific gravity
SHO	Senior House Officer (UK)
SI	sacro-iliac
sig.	label (in prescriptions)
s.l.	sublingual
SM	systolic murmur
SMR	sub-mucous resection
SN	student nurse (UK)
SOB	short of breath
SOBOE	short of breath on exertion
SOP	surgical out-patients
SRN	State Registered Nurse (UK)
SROM	spontaneous rupture of membranes
ST's	sanitary towels
SVC	superior vena cava
SVD	simple vertex delivery
SWD	short wave diathermy

T	temperature
tabs	tablets
T & A	tonsils and adenoids
TB	tuberculosis
t.d.s./t.i.d.	three times daily
TI	tricuspid incompetence
TIA	transient isotemic attack
TMJ	temporo mandibular joint
TNS	transcutaneous nerve stimulator
TOP	treponemal immobilisation test
TPR	temperature, pulse, respiration
TR	temporary resident (UK)
TS	tricuspid stenosis
TT	tetanus toxoid; tuberculin tested
TV	trichomonas vaginalis
TUR	transurethral prostate resection

U	urea
U & E	urea and electrolytes
UGS	urogenital system
UMN	upper motor neurone
URTI	upper respiratory tract infection
USP	United States Pharmacopeic
UVL	ultra-violet light

VD	venereal disease
VDRL	venereal disease research laboratory
VE	vaginal examination
VI	virgo intacta
VP	venous pressure
VSD	ventricular septal defect
VV	varicose vein(s)
Vx	vertex

W	widow/widower
WBC	white blood cell count; white blood corpuscles
WNL	within normal limits
WR	Wassermann reaction
XR	X-ray
YOB	year of birth

Appendix 3   Who's who in the British hospital system

CONSULTANT
The most senior position held by physicians or surgeons with the highest qualifications e.g. FRCS MRCP*.

MEDICAL ASSISTANT
A senior position held by a doctor with many years experience but without a higher qualification.

SENIOR REGISTRAR
A position held by a doctor with the highest degree in a chosen speciality, two years experience in a general hospital, and two years experience in the chosen speciality in a teaching hospital*.

REGISTRAR
A position held by a doctor who usually has a higher qualification.

SENIOR HOUSE OFFICER
A one year appointment (usually residential) held by a doctor who is studying for a higher qualification.

HOUSE OFFICER
A position held by a doctor who has completed the pre-registration year.

PRE-REGISTRATION HOUSE OFFICER
A position held by a newly qualified doctor for one year, prior to full registration.

DIRECTOR OF NURSING SERVICES
The most senior position in nursing administration.

SENIOR NURSE
A senior management position.

DEPARTMENTAL SISTER
A senior position for a nurse with experience and either SRN or RGN (three years training).

WARD SISTER
A qualified and experienced nurse with overall responsibility for a ward.

STAFF NURSE
First post for a SRN/RGN qualified nurse.

STATE ENROLLED NURSE
A post held by a nurse who has completed the short two year training course.

NURSING AUXILIARY / NURSING ASSISTANT
Untrained nursing assistants.

* Note that Consultants and Senior Registrars who are surgeons drop the title Dr and are addressed as Mr/Mrs/Ms/Miss.

Appendix 4   A broad equivalence of positions in the NHS and the US hospital systems

NHS	UK University	US Hospital	US University
Consultant	Senior Lecturer / Professor	Attending Physician	Fellow / Associate Professor
*Senior Registrar	Lecturer	*Senior Resident	Assistant
Registrar	Lecturer	Resident (Year 2/3)	Assistant
Senior House Officer	—	Resident (Year 1)	—
House Officer	—	Interne	—

* In the UK a Senior Registrar may hold the post for 4 years whereas in the US a Senior Resident does only one year.

Appendix 5   Useful addresses

British

British Medical Association
BMA House
Tavistock Square
London WC1H 9JR

Council for Postgraduate Medical Education in England and Wales
7 Marylebone Road
London NW1 5HH

Department of Health and Social Security
Alexander Fleming House
Newington Causeway
Elephant and Castle
London SE1 6BY

General Medical Council
44 Hallam Street
London W1N 6AE

General Medical Council
Overseas Registration Division
153 Cleveland Street
London W1P 6DE

General Nursing Council for England and Wales
23 Portland Place
London W1N 4DE

General Nursing Council for Scotland
5 Darnaway Street
Edinburgh EH3 6DP

Medical Defence Union
3 Devonshire Place
London W1N 2EA

Medical and Dental Union of Scotland
113 St Vincent Street
Glasgow G2 5EQ

Medical Practitioners' Union
79 Camden Road
London NW1 9ES

Medical Protection Society
50 Hallam Street
London W1N 6DE

Medical Research Council
20 Park Crescent
London W1N 4AL

Royal College of General Practitioners
14 Princes Gate
Hyde Park
London SW7 1PU

Royal College of Midwives
15 Mansfield Street
London W1M 0BE

The Royal College of Physicians of London
11 St Andrews Place
Regents Park
London NW1 4LE

The Royal College of Surgeons of England
35–43 Lincoln's Inn Fields
London WC2A 3PN

American

American Medical Association
535 N Dearborn Street
Chicago IL 60610

American Academy of Family Physicians
1740 W 92nd Street
Kansas City MO 64114

American College of Physicians
4200 Pine Street
Philadelphia PA 19104

American College of Surgeons
55 E Erie Street
Chicago IL 60611

American Federation for Clinical Research
University of Washington
Children's Orthopedic Hospital and Medical Center
PO Box C–5371 Seattle WA 98105

American Hospital Association
Intermountain Health Center Inc.
36 S State Street
Salt Lake City UT 84111

Educational Commission for Foreign Medical Graduates
3624 Market Street
Philadelphia PENN 19104–2685

Southern Medical Association
35 Lakeshore Drive
PO Box 63656 Birmingham AL 35219–0088

Acknowledgements

The authors and publishers are grateful to the following for permission to reproduce copyright material:

p. 14, Update Publications Ltd for E. R. Beck *et al.,* 'Two cases of pneumonia', *Hospital Update,* January 1977, p. 43; **p. 27,** McGraw-Hill Book Company for R. G. Petersdorf *et al., Harrison's Principles of Internal Medicine,* 10th edn, 1983, pp. 1425–6, 1459; **pp. 36–7,** British Medical Association/The Pharmaceutical Society of Great Britain for extracts from the *British National Formulary,* 11, A. Prasad (ed.), London, 1986, pp. 189–208; **pp. 48–50,** *Archives of Internal Medicine* for T. Nakamura *et al.,* 'Iatronic areteriovenous fistula of the internal mammary artery', vol. 145, January 1985, pp. 140–1, © 1985, American Medical Association; **p. 61,** British Medical Association for J. W. Howie, 'How I read', *British Medical Journal,* vol. 3, 1976, p. 1125; **pp. 62–3,** British Medical Association for D. R. Naik *et al.,* 'Comparison of barium swallow and ultrasound in diagnosis of gastro-oesophageal reflux in children', *British Medical Journal,* vol. 290, 1985, pp. 1943–5; **p. 70,** Churchill-Livingstone for J. C. Adams, *Outline of Orthopaedics,* 10th edn, 1986, p. 217; **pp. 72–4,** British Medical Association for J. Curran *et al.,* 'Practice of preoperative assessment by anaesthetists', *British Medical Journal,* vol. 291, 1985, pp. 391–3; **pp. 86–8,** extracts from *Current Contents®,* vol. 27, 25, June 18, 1984, reprinted with permission and copyright owned by the Institute for Scientific Information®, Philadelphia, USA: **p. 89,** Contents Page, *Transplantation,* vol. 37, 5, © by Williams and Wilkins, 1984; **p. 90,** J. W. Alexander *et al.,* 'The late adverse effect of splenectomy on patient survival following cadaveric renal transplantation', *Transplantation;* **p. 91,** T. Tamura *et al.,* 'Specificity of transplantation heterophile antibodies', *Transplantation;* **p. 91,** M. I. Koolen *et al.,* 'Excretion of urokallikrein in renal transplant patients', *Transplantation;* **p. 90,** S. Karger AG, Basel for M. R. Berk *et al.,* 'Non-typhoid salmonella infections after renal transplantation', *Nephron,* vol. 37, 1984, p. 186.

Book design and artwork by Hobson Street Studio, Cambridge